The Prince

and the

Caregiver

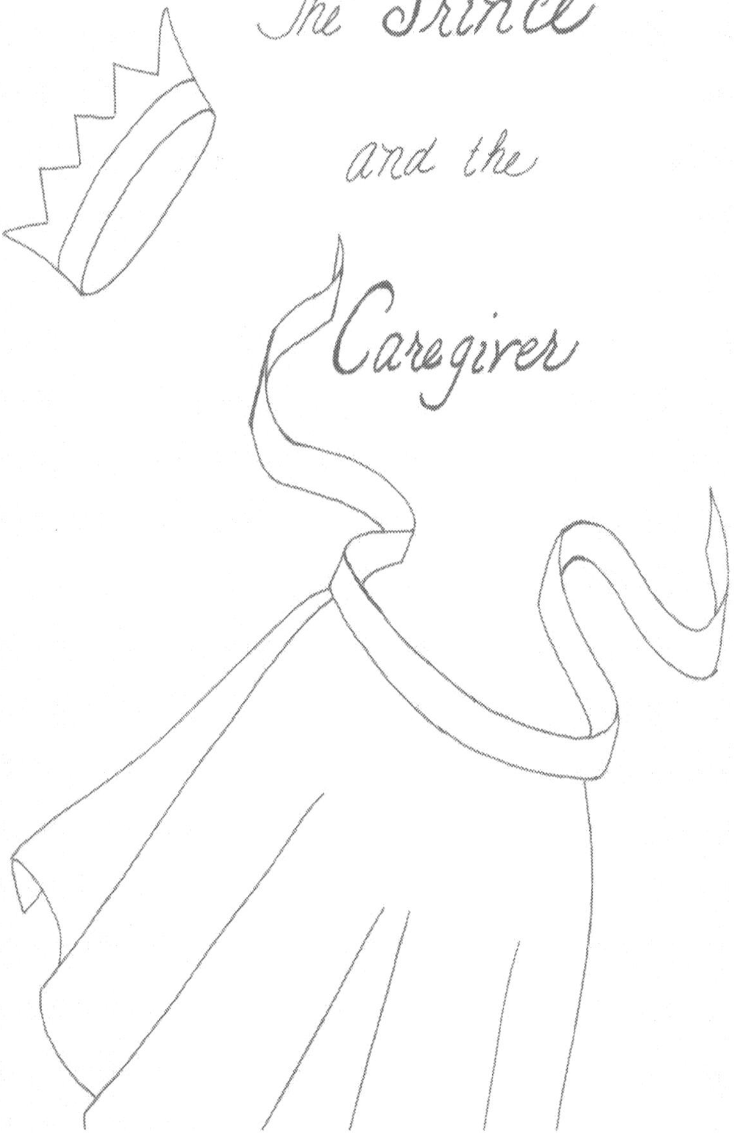

Written By Maureen A. Schulz

Illustrated By Betsy Reif

First published by AuthorHouse 04/20/04

ISBN: 1-4140-5694-X (e-book)
ISBN: 1-4184-4498-7 (Paperback)

Library of Congress Control Number: 2003099936

This book is printed on acid free paper.

Printed in the United States of America
Bloomington, IN

Special thanks to all my many friends who helped in this project in any way.

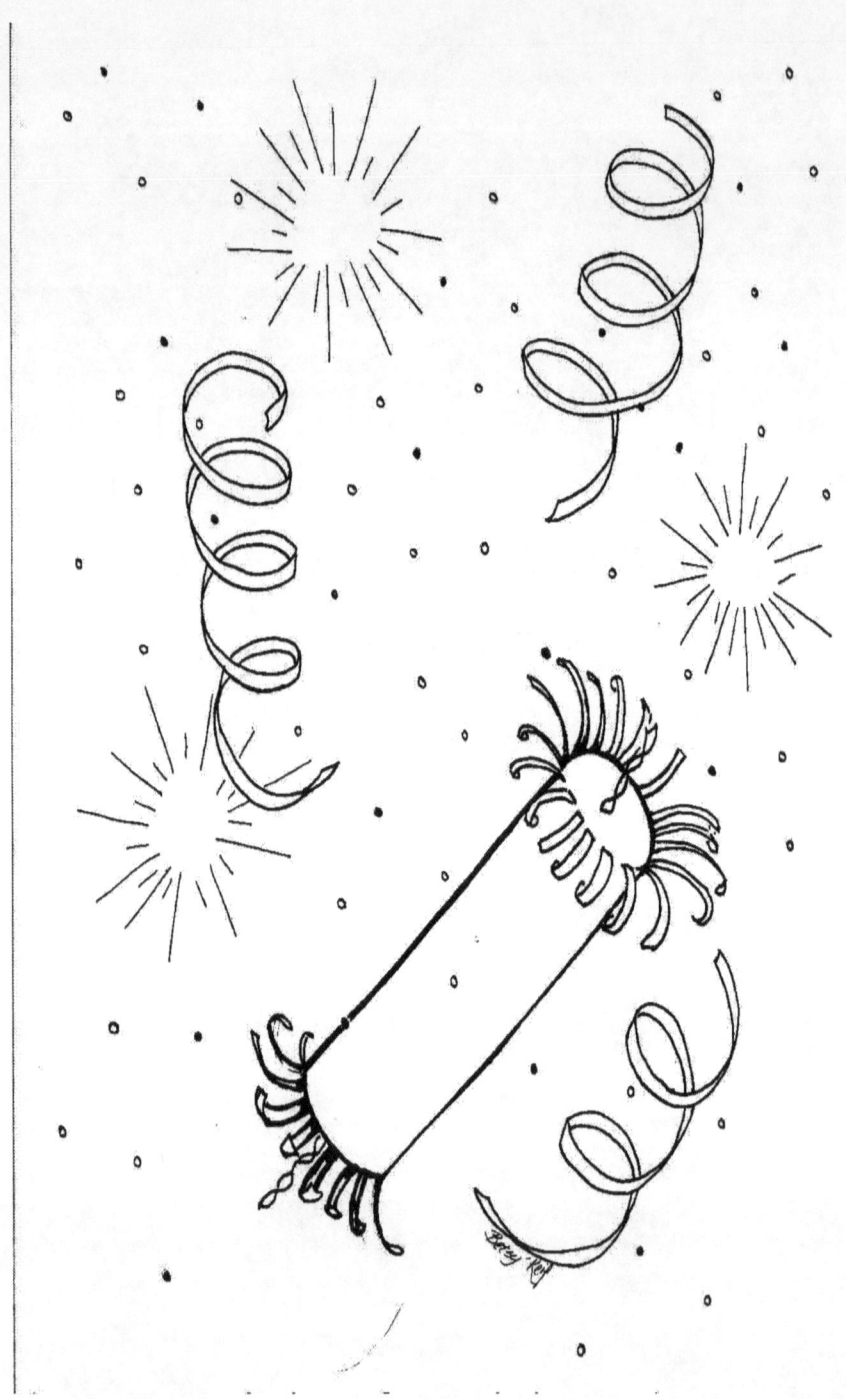

Chapter One

I Meet My Prince

"And the king loved Esther above all women, and she obtained grace and favour in his sight more than all the virgins so that he set the royal crown upon her head, and made her queen..." Esther 2:17

Jerry and I met on December 31, 1968, at nine o'clock in the evening. There are certain dates and hours that we cannot forget-when we accept Jesus as Lord and Savior and are Born Again, when we are baptized in the Holy Spirit with the evidence of speaking in tongues, the births of children, marriages, and deaths.

In my life, my first meeting with my future husband, my prince, ranks along with the other important moments in my life. Neither of us was saved and we were leading worldly lives. As you can tell by the date, it was New Year's Eve. It was also a blind date set up by his first wife's family.

Evon, his first wife, had been killed in a car accident two years earlier.

The family took us to some animal club- Moose, Elks, Lions or something, in Deadwood, South Dakota. At midnight, we kissed amid horns, noisemakers, and cheering. He looked deep into my eyes and asked me to marry him. To my utter shock, I heard myself saying "yes". I thought to myself, just wait until tomorrow when this guy realizes what he just did. I'll never see him again. Once more, I reminded myself, I don't like blind dates and I will never go on another one. Marriage was definitely not on my agenda.

After that first kiss, I found myself wondering just how much he had been drinking before he picked me up for the date. He had only had one drink that I knew about. I wondered if he would even remember that proposal the next day. Well, he not only remembered it, he repeated it. I thought he was nuts.

Jerry was a big man, six foot tall and muscular. His hair was thinning on top and he had the most beautiful blue eyes. He never thought he could sing but, oh, how he could whistle, melody after melody of beautiful music. He was my gentle giant but I didn't realize it for many years. Because of my first marriage, I was almost afraid of him because of his size when we first met. But his gentleness won me over in no time at all.

I was a divorced mother of two, in my senior year of college, and I had no plans to marry again. I had two part-time jobs, two children, a house to take care of, and I usually carried an overload of college credits. Marriage was not for me. I didn't want to let some man have any rights over my children or me. I didn't want to be another alcoholic man's punching bag, which was why I divorced in the first place.

My dating in college was practically non-existent. I usually went out with a group or would meet up with a group off-campus. I had one rule that I very seldom broke and that was to take my own car.

The first year, I was drinking a lot. My children were staying with my parents and I was lonesome for my children. I didn't have a car (which was a very good thing, considering how much I was drinking) so that year the rule was to stay with a group. There was safety in numbers.

I could not believe that I would say "yes" to a marriage proposal from some guy I had just met. I lived in Spearfish, South Dakota, and he lived in Milwaukee, Wisconsin. He was in South Dakota on vacation to see his young son who was living with his mother's relatives. Again I thought, after this guy goes back to Wisconsin, I'll never hear from him again. I was wrong.

Jerry started a barrage of telephone calls, usually timed when I would be home from work. We conducted a long-distance romance and Ma Bell was our chaperon. Actually, we got to know one another through discussions without the turmoil and stress of being face to face, necking, touching, wondering what to wear, where to go, showing someone you like them without loosing their respect. Perhaps there is something to be said for arranged marriages, chaperons, and their place in life.

I went to Wisconsin in mid-March to interview for jobs. At that time, he gave me a beautiful diamond engagement ring. I didn't find a job at that time, but we set our wedding plans. We would get married on May 27, 1969, at seven, in the Lutheran church. We did marry on May 27, 1969, but at five o'clock in the evening, and we went to Sundance, Wyoming, and married before a Justice of the Peace. We spent a week together before he had to go back to work. It was mid-July before I was able to go to Wisconsin.

It was a little stressful trying to integrate two households together. Jerry had a twelve-year-old son, Steve, and a ten-year-old dog. I had an eight-year-old daughter, Lila, a six year old, Jerry Lee, a gad about a dog and a cross-eyed cat. At times it felt like Noah's Ark.

And then there were the doubles. We had two toasters, two irons, two sewing machines, two vacuum cleaners, etc. I always intended to have a yard sale but, somehow, never did. It took years to wear out all that stuff.

Speaking of Noah's Ark (Gen. Chapters six through nine) and the two by two's, did you ever stop to think what it must been like? First of all, it had never rained on the earth before. God watered the earth with dew every night (Gen. 2:6). So there was a host of new words and ideas like rain, storm, lightning, thunder, flood, and ark. It took one hundred years, but Noah had to built an ark like God told him- 450 feet long, 75 feet wide, and 45 feet high, it had three floors, one door and one window. It would be claustrophobic, dark, and with all those animals noisy and smelly.

On vacation one year, in Florida, we camped overnight with a tent camper in the parking lot at the Ft. Lauderdale Lion Country Safari. It was extremely noisy with all those elephants trumpeting, peacocks shrieking, lions and all the big cats roaring all night long. No one was able to sleep with animals just behind a fence. The kids were afraid to sleep and were asking all night long, "What was that?" and "Are you sure they can't get through that fence?" I didn't get to sleep much either. After all, someone had to stay awake and answer their questions.

How Mr. Noah and his sons ever talked those women into getting into that ark, I can't imagine, especially with all those mice, rats, bugs, and snakes. You don't think so? Check Gen. 7:8. I can just imagine Mrs. Noah telling him "You let those animals in so you go feed them and clean up after them. I'm not going down there." You don't think he had a time of it? The second thing he did when he stepped out on terra firma was plant a vineyard and get drunk (Gen. 9:20-21). Think it's not so? Keep on reading!

And it was deep! There were twenty-one feet and six inches of water over the tops of the mountains. And it was months and months and months of nothing but water, water, water...

And where was God in all of this? Inside. How do you know for sure? By what God said. Twice God said, "Come into the ark." Not "Go into the ark." He was inside and bade them to come on in. Then there are all the symbolic things about the ark. Inside with God was protection and life. It wasn't dark. He is the light of the world and where he is there is no darkness found. God caused it to be filled with

5

fresh air and comfortable temperatures. It doesn't tell about them taking provisions on board for people AND creatures. As big as it was and with all those animals I believe that God cared for the creatures. And Mrs. Noah didn't say a word. They were ALL cared for and fed.

God made a covenant with Noah (Gen. 6:18) that was a covenant of protection and safety from another earth-covering flood, and the sign of it was a rainbow (Gen. 9:12-17). The first thing Noah did was to build an altar and offered burnt offerings (Gen. 8:20). The second thing he did was plant a vineyard. Some animals did NOT go in two by two but in sevens (Gen. 7:2) because Noah would have to make an offering to God from the clean animals that landed.

Remember when I talked about Mrs. Noah and the girls? Well, you just remember that things go smoothly when God is the head of the family, in every room of the house (or heart), and in every situation. It's true. Things go better with God.

I started teaching that fall and our lives fell into pattern. I took ceramic classes and Jerry took them, also. One spring evening, just before school was out, we were at ceramics class and I was writing out a check. Suddenly, I gasped and started to laugh. Everyone wanted to know what was the matter. Jerry even asked me if we were overdrawn. "No," I laughed. "I just realized what today is. It's our anniversary." Amid choruses of "Happy Anniversary", someone finally asked, "Which one?"

In a very small, quiet voice, I answered, "The first." Everyone laughed hilariously that we had forgotten our first anniversary. But we were comfortable, spending quality time and doing many projects, together. However, Jerry must have thought something was wrong because he never forgot another wedding anniversary. He never forgot birthdays, the anniversary of the day we met, first kiss, Sweetest Day, Valentine's Day, Mother's Day, or any other day that was a good excuse to celebrate something.

Jerry loved people and being around them. He always made people feel at ease and was a wonderful host. He had a tremendous sense of humor and a million jokes. I always thought we should have written his jokes down into a book. Not only were they funny but after he was saved, they were clean jokes you could tell anyone. We even had doctors call up and say, "Jerry, give me a joke, quick. I've got to speak at a meeting tonight and I need a joke to break the ice." That was his reputation among the people with whom he came in contact.

Jerry was an avid golfer. Our second summer, he complained of his shoulder hurting until he finally agreed to go to the doctor. The doctor said he had a 'tennis elbow' type of injury to the shoulder and gave him cortisone shots to ease the pain. The shots hurt like blazes but, afterward, he felt so good that he even talked me into trying to learn golf. More quality time we were spending together. Life was good. We bowled in the wintertime on bowling leagues, continued our ceramics classes, entering contests, tournaments, and started art classes.

After our second wedding anniversary, after school was out, I started to notice how much Jerry was drinking, soft drinks, alcohol, mixes, milk, Koolaid, everything and anything. His thirst was insatiable. But what bothered me was the amount of alcohol he was consuming. He was drinking a fifth of whiskey, every two days, in mixed drinks. Finally, I couldn't take it any more. I said, "I was married to one alcoholic and I will not live with another."

He said, "I'll quit. I don't need the alcohol. I just need something cold to drink." He immediately quit drinking alcohol at home but he was still drinking enormous amount of cold liquids. It bothered me but I didn't know anything was physically wrong with him. I didn't know anything at all about sugar diabetes let alone what the warning signs of the disease were.

We had been married two and a half years when we attended a Halloween party with the family, friends, and kids in tow. Jerry had a few drinks over the next five or six hours, but not enough to worry me with all the food and snacks he was eating. On the way home, his voice started to slur and he began passing out for a second or two and then coming to again. I was scared but he assured me that he was all right. Suddenly he stiffened out with his head back and his foot on the gas pedal but he dropped his hand from the steering wheel.

"Steve," I yelled, "steer the car!" I got down on the floor of the car, first to try to get to the brake, and when that failed, to try to get Jerry's foot off the gas pedal. I finally succeeded, and we got the car stopped on the shoulder of the road. I turned it off and took the keys. At last, with all doors open, he started to come around. At first, he didn't know where he was or what had happened. I was very, very frightened and so were the kids.

We went home, and I argued with him to go to the hospital to be checked. I was afraid of a heart attack because he had told me that his mother had died in her forties of a heart attack. He finally agreed and we called the hospital to tell them we were coming. We left the kids at home and went to the emergency room. They decided he had not had a heart attack but they didn't know what was going on. I gave them his medical history that I knew, which wasn't much. I went home and the next day I called his sister to ask her the questions that the doctor had asked me about what kinds of illnesses were in his family history. That's when I found out that his grandmother and some aunts had died of diabetes.

They kept him for a week and we had appointments to see doctors. They started him on pills. They told us he had too much sugar in his blood. And they told us that the pills would take the sugar out of his blood. And they told us he had diabetes. It was one of the reasons he decided that he didn't want any more children. Several years later we were told that a cortisone shot could bring out diabetes in the borderline diabetic. It was less than six months since he had gotten the cortisone shot.

The dying had begun.

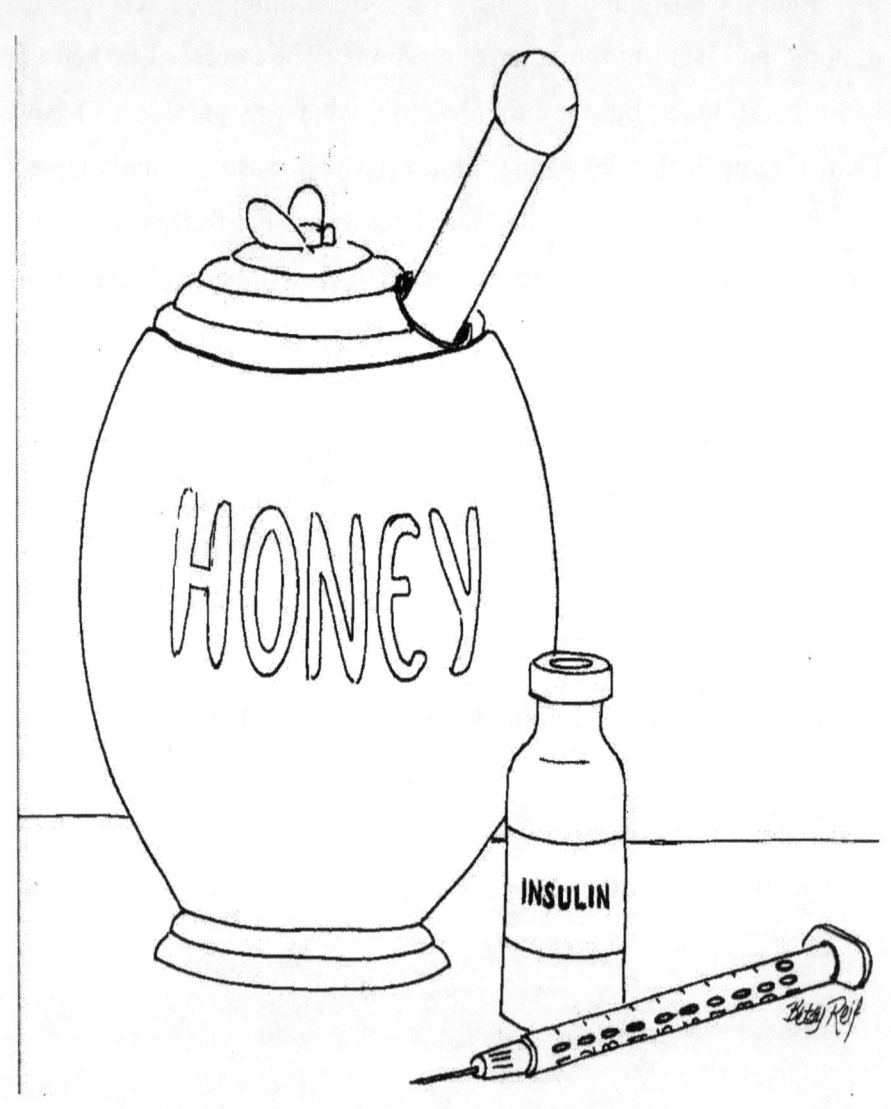

Chapter Two

John Wayne, Dustin Hoffman, Robin Williams

"And the Lord God commanded the man saying, of every tree of the garden thou mayest freely eat: but of the tree of the knowledge of good and evil, thou shall not eat of it: for in the day that thou eatest thereof thou shalt surely die: Gen. 2:16-17

I loved my husband. Like John Wayne, he was tall and good-looking, with a killer smile and his eyes were the most beautiful shade of blue. Like Dustin Hoffman, he was very sensitive, and when he was hurt or sad, my sensitive husband could cry. (Real men CAN cry and do.) Like Robin Williams, he had a terrific sense of humor, enjoying making other people laugh and feel at ease.

Jerry and I had many trials trying to put two families together. The kids didn't like each other, the dogs didn't like each other, the cat didn't like anything, and Jerry and I were still trying to learn about each other. There was a lot we didn't know since our romance had been carried on over long distance lines with Ma Bell as a chaperone. But we were both very determined to make it work.

One of the first things we were told about his diabetes was that if he ever ran OUT of or LOW on the blood sugar, he should eat honey. It had already been digested by bees, and would get into the bloodstream faster. Jerry always had to carry a packet of honey everywhere, his locker at work, golf bag, glove compartment of the car, and his pocket, whenever he felt faint he was to eat some honey.

This is backed up by Scripture. I Sam. 13 tells about Saul and his army getting ready to go to battle. I Sam. 14:24 tells how the Israelites were hard pressed and King Saul had forbidden the army to even taste of food. But God prepared food for them. He covered the floor of the forest with honey because they needed the blood sugar. But the army could not eat any because the king had promised death to any one who did. But his son, Jonathon and Jonathon's armor bearer, did not hear the king. So they ate, went into their own battle and won.

When Jonathon returned, he saw the army had not eaten the honey and had done poorly against the enemy. Jonathon said that his father had troubled the land. Jonathon said his own eyes were brightened because he ate the honey and, if the army had eaten, they would have made a great slaughter against the enemy. I Sam. 14:32 tells how the army fell on the spoils, took the animals and ate them raw, thus committing sin by eating the meat with the blood. King Saul made the people sin by not letting them eat the perfect food, honey, that God had provided. When Saul learned that his own son had eaten honey, lots were cast and he was ready to have Jonathon killed. But the people themselves said that Jonathon had delivered them from the enemy and should not die (I Sam. 14:46).

The diabetes was hard to get a handle on at first. It seemed as if the doctors were learning about it just as we were. At first, he was told to take some little white pills and then some stronger little blue ones. Then he wound up in the hospital for a week. The new doctor said not to take any more of those pills. They take the sugar OUT of your system. You are running OUT of sugar without the pills. You don't need them. It's still diabetes, but the form YOU have is hypoglycemia. At first I tried to read everything I could find on diabetes. We were sure that if we tried hard enough we could beat it or at least control it. It never seemed possible that it would control us.

The year following Jerry's diagnosis, I quit teaching. I got another job closer to the house. I was elected Town Clerk. My husband supported me, helped me many times, (not quite Mr. Mom but very helpful) and we continued to learn about diabetes. I could come home for lunch and, since Jerry worked second shift, it gave us some time together. I could make sure he ate properly. Then he started to pick me up at work and take me out for lunch. I let him. It was easier than arguing about it, especially when he said he was doing it to spend more time with me and to be good to me. And he always knew that he could get away with it. I did not like arguments and would never argue with him in public. He would give the waitress his order and look at me as if to dare me say anything. Sometimes, I would just say, "It's your body," and his immediate comeback would be, "That's right." At one point, he started to pick me up after work and go to visit his sister just in time for supper because at her house he would eat as much and whatever he wanted and I would be quiet about it.

Jerry had diabetic ulcers on his legs and a few on his face that were very hard to heal. In fact, one doctor asked him if he had been a hockey player because of the scars on his legs.

We received advice from EVERYONE about how to heal the ulcers. One of the benefits of living in a small town is that everyone knows all about everyone else. We learned about all the diabetics in everyone's families and all the things they did with any degree of success. We heard all kinds of hair-brained-ideas- from applying raw onions, potato, lemon, apple, beet, kiwi slices, to bandages soaked with everything from vinegar to sugar water. I heard about hot and cold poultices made with everything from garlic mustard to chopped alfalfa.

One well meaning lady told us we could totally cure his diabetes if he would just drink three big glasses of yellow water- just plain yellow food coloring and plain water- every day for two weeks and longer if necessary. We discussed them all, went home determined to stick closely to what the doctors prescribed. They had studied many years and were supposed to know what they were talking about. At any rate, Jerry told me he had received many warnings from early childhood on not to eat any yellow snow and thereof, he elected to pass on the yellow water, also.

14

At this time, while I am telling you about the type of advice we received, especially from worldly people, I must tell you about two women who TRULY were helpful but from a much later time period.

At this time, Jerry had been a diabetic twenty-one years, was blind, in a wheelchair, incontinent and required a great deal of care, when my doctor bullied me into having a mammogram. I didn't like them and hadn't had one in fifteen years. They found a lump. I had to have surgery. I tried everywhere to find someone who would take care of Jerry. I postponed my surgery twice, and the doctor was getting upset with me, but I couldn't find anyone who was willing to care for him.

I called home health agencies but for someone to take care of him for that long, it would have to be ordered by one of HIS doctors. And it was too expensive for me to pay for the service. Finally, my cousin from northeast of Dallas called and as we talked, she offered to come and stay for a while. I had two days to teach her how to give insulin shots, change condom catheters, and take care of Jerry's sores, etc. Now, she could stay with Jerry while I had my surgery but she didn't know the city and I still needed someone to take me to the hospital and bring me home afterward, as they didn't want me to drive myself.

I remembered a woman, a total stranger, I had met in a church, gave me her telephone number and told me that if I ever needed help I should just ask. So I asked. This wonderful woman had me at the hospital at seven a.m. and then STAYED with me all day. She prayed with me before the surgery, and throughout the day, she called my house to report to Jerry and my cousin what was happening. Jerry was very worried about me. I was finally allowed to come home about six p.m. and this wonderful lady even stopped at a pharmacy to get my prescriptions filled. She even got them filled and paid for them while I waited in her van.

My cousin then stayed with me for two weeks because the doctors said I was not to lift anything heavy (like Jerry's wheelchair in and out of the car or helping Jerry move in an out of bed, toilet, car, wheelchair, couch, or anywhere). I thanked those two women and I thank God for them. When I remembered the story of the Good Samaritan, I always think of them. Most people, when you ask for help, will give an excuse of why they can't. VERY few people will respond with, "What do you need and when do you need it?" And they did not expect nor would they accept payment. God bless you both, forever and ever. May God repay you out of His bountiful blessings. Very, very few people are willing to help or get involved. But this happened many years later after we had moved to Texas.

Meanwhile, back at beginning, I had to take several nutrition classes and cooking classes at he hospital. The idea was that his diabetes could, at this point, be diet-controlled. We made the whole family eat this nutritious diet. Only Jerry's food was measured by the ounce.

About this time, I joined weight loss class. I continued to cook meals for the rest of the family while I cooked for myself one hotdog-slit in half, on a slice of white bread-very carefully sliced into two slices, (to fool your mind into believing there was more food on the plate than there really was), with mustard, plain lettuce and skim milk. Ta Daa! Dinner is served. One thing I learned at this time was that you can fool your eye but you cannot fool your stomach.

After about three weeks of me being on MY diet, Jerry came up behind me while I was at the stove. He slid his arms around me and asked, "Where did you ever get the idea you are too fat?" He shut off all the burners and said, "I'm tired of this stuff. We're going out for pizza." It was the beginning of a long and close relationship with the lady at the pizzeria. It was also the end of my dieting. I had not realized how horribly grouchy I was while trying to diet. I was trying to diet hoping to look better. Jerry's diet was hopefully to give better quality and extension to his life.

One of the other patrons of the pizzeria was also a diabetic and I wondered how he could eat everything he seemed to want with no ill effects on his health. He also claimed to be diet controlled with no pills or shots. We went to his doctor and we were helped a lot. Now, Jerry's diabetes was also diet controlled. But Jerry also liked to treat himself. The doctors called it cheating on his diet. I won't tell you what I called it. At work and on the way home from work he would eat all the things that he wanted that were not on his diet. Doctors would come down on me for not keeping him on his diet.

At first I didn't understand what was going on, how his sugar could be so high while he was on this diet. He didn't like saccharine or any of the sweeteners that leave an after taste. I tried some of the sugar free of low sugar desserts. There were very few that he would eat. The hospitals would give us recipes and meal planning books with all the diabetic exchanges in them. I finally realized, after he became legally blind, just how much he had been cheating on his diet. I had to do all the driving and take him wherever he wanted to go, like the local ice cream stand. He had to eat meals at home-no more stopping on the way home for pie, cake, donuts, pastries, sandwiches, etc.

I wanted him to stay on the diet that he hated so much, so that he would live longer and have a better quality of life, that he would be with me and we would happily grow old together-only he wasn't happy. He said he knew that he would live longer eating only from the diabetic diet, but he had no enjoyment eating only food that he did not like.

Jerry did not like the feeling that he was not in control of his own life. He continued to burn the candle on both ends giving up sleep to play golf or do something he wanted rather than get rest. This was hard on him. He had to work second shift, or, as I used to call it, second and a half shift because he started at eight o'clock at night and worked until five o'clock the next morning. However, when we were first married, he would often have to work straight through double and triple shifts with no breaks at all for rest.

There were times he would tell me that he couldn't sleep because it was too noisy in the house. So I would take the kids and leave for the day. That meant I didn't get to do a lot of the housework big jobs-things you leave for the weekend- and that would leave me frustrated and cranky.

Just like Adam and Eve with the apple, he would do as he wanted, satisfy his desires and eat the foods that he knew were bad for him, and would certainly kill him physically in the end.

The demon of diabetes was gaining ground.

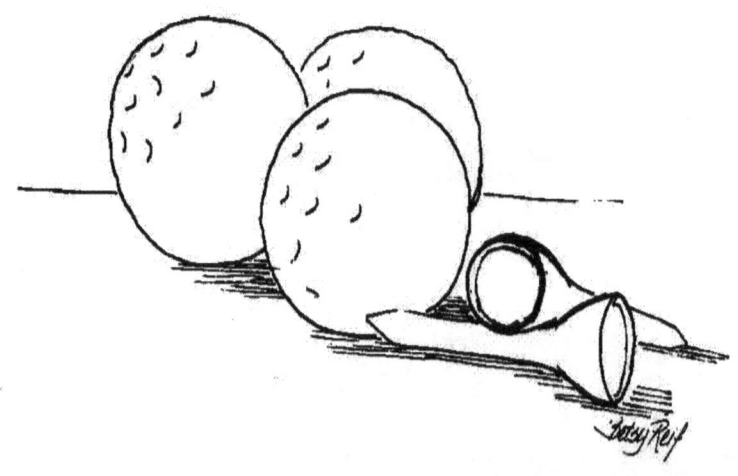

Chapter Three

A Man With A Merry Heart

Jerry's joke for this section.

> Jesus, Moses and an older fellow went out to play golf.
> Moses hit the first ball and it went in the water. Moses parted the water and retrieved his ball. Jesus hit the next ball and it went in the water also, so He walked on the water and retrieved His ball.
> The older fellow hit his ball and it skipped across the water, flew across the green, hit a tree, came back on the green, circle the cup three times and finally rolled in.
> Jesus looked at Moses, shrugged His shoulders and looked at the older fellow and said, "Nice shot, Dad."

One of our Christian friends heard this joke from Jerry, said he was blaspheming and committing an unforgivable sin. So Jerry didn't tell ANY jokes at all for about six months. I tried to tell him it was not blasphemy but the Christian friend was older; Jerry greatly respected his advice and teaching, receiving the admonition as gospel.

Jerry started to decline. There was just no other word for it. He did not laugh or smile. He wouldn't think of saying anything funny, let alone tell a joke. My funny, merry-hearted husband turned into the worst Gloomy Gus you can imagine.

I finally took him to our pastor and told him what had happened. I asked Pastor Wayne if his joke was blaspheming. He laughed at the joke and assured us it was not blaspheming. Then Pastor Wayne told us a similar joke involving tennis, which was his game. I don't remember all of the joke, I just know you can never win a tennis match playing against God because He always starts with love.

This is an important lesson. Don't let anybody, I mean ANYBODY, mess with your loved one's head. Or yours. Well-meaning Christians and even pastors, who should know better, say a lot of things that are better left unsaid. A person who does not know the Word of God is vulnerable to "Super Saints", "God Cops", and "Gospel Deputies". Those people who sometimes don't rightly divide the word of God but try to teach, anyway. Three of the gospels, Mathew, Mark, and Luke, teach on this subject, quoting Jesus:

3. (Jesus) said, Truly I say to you, unless you repent (change, turn around) and become like little children [trusting, lowly, loving, forgiving) you can never enter the kingdom of heaven at all.

4. Whoever will humble himself therefore, and becomes [trusting, lowly, loving, forgiving) as this little child, is the greatest in the kingdom of heaven;

5. And whoever receives and accepts and welcomes one little child like this for My sake and in My name receives and accepts and welcomes Me.

6. But whoever causes one of these little ones who believe in and acknowledge and cleave to Me to stumble and sin- that is, who entices him, or hinders him in right conduct or thought- it would be better (more expedient and profitable or advantageous) for him to have a great millstone fastened around his neck and to be sunk in the depth of the sea. (Mt. 18:3-6 Amp)

In Jerry's case, he looked up to a Bible Study teacher taking a criticism from that person to heart. He wound up declining and getting worse because he stopped telling jokes and gave up something in his life that gave him joy. The Bible says that, "A merry heart doeth good like a medicine: but a broken spirit drieth the bones" (Prov. 17:22). I saw this actually happening.

After talking to the Pastor about what constituted blasphemy and what was not blasphemy, my funny, merry hearted husband began telling jokes again. He had joy back in his soul. He got healthier and felt better. I did, too. Besides, I liked his jokes.

This is something for the Super Saints, God Cops, and Gospel Deputies to study:

> Truly and solemnly I say to you, all sins will be forgiven the sons of men, and whatever abusive and blasphemous things they utter;
> But whoever speaks abusively against or maliciously misrepresents the Holy Spirit can never get forgiveness, but is guilty of and is in the grasp of an everlasting trespass. (M'r 3:28-29, Amp.)

That is what blasphemy is: abusively or maliciously misrepresenting the Holy Spirit. I PERSONALLY believe that this also means to ATTRIBUTE the WORKS of the Holy Spirit to Satan. I guess that would be considered malicious.

For anyone who is not familiar with a millstone, it works the same as a cement block and does not float. The Mafia is reputed to have used this procedure effectively in the past.

A few years later, a pastor took Jerry to task. It seemed he was not "politically correct" in some of his jokes. So we changed them so he could tell them without offending anyone.

Worldly people and complete strangers can and do hurt your patient by things they say and do. In Milwaukee, Jerry liked to ride the bus after he could not drive anymore. He enjoyed hearing the names of the stops the driver called out. He could see good enough to walk to the bus stop and the driver soon became acquainted with him.

One day he fell while waiting for the bus. High school students were sitting on the bench and Jerry had to wait standing up. His legs gave out and he couldn't get up. They started laughing and jeering at him. They said he was drunk and started laughing at him and spitting on him. The bus came and the driver helped him over to sit on the bench. Jerry said he didn't want to go on the bus anymore. He would just rest and go home.

We went to a drug store one day and I pushed Jerry in his wheelchair and he would hold the small carrying basket. I parked him behind another shopping cart that had a small child in it. Because he was almost blind, I told Jerry there was a cart ahead of us with a toddler in it. He started to wiggle his fingers and wave at the child. I went down the isle and he stayed behind the cart. I wasn't there when the mother came back and called him a "Pervert" for attempting to play with the child. He demanded to leave the store immediately and we were in the car before he would tell me what had happened.

This was the man who liked kids and enjoyed working in Children's Church. Every summer our whole church took a week and went camping at Family Camp, but we were only able to go once, but that once was when he had over a hundred kids who were calling him "Grandpa Jerry".

In wasn't just strangers, either. The son of a neighbor down the street going to elementary school would stop and say hello to Jerry when he sat outside. After Jerry told the youngster he was blind, Jason would always stop and ask how he was doing. Jason would shake Jerry's hand and tell Jerry, "Hi, Jerry, it's Jason," letting Jerry know who was speaking. He would sit for a few minutes and Jerry would ask what he doing in school, etc.

Jason and his manners impressed Jerry and he said he wanted to stop and tell Jason's parents what a nice young man they were raising. I had a check in my spirit but Jerry insisted. We stopped and told them what a nice boy Jason was. He never stopped or said "Hi," again. I always wondered if he was punished for not going straight home after school. He would almost seem to want to run past our house. He never stopped to speak to Jerry again.

A joke from Jerry to lighten things up and change the subject.

> Do you know how nacho cheese got its name? No? Well there was this hippie who went to the food pantry and on the top of the sack there was five pounds of cheese. As he was walking away, another guy runs by and grabs the cheese. The hippie yells after him, "Hey, man! That's not cho' cheese!"

If you are a caregiver, involved in special diets and foods, invest right away in cookbooks regarding that patient's nutritional needs, especially those written with the particular health problem in mind. You know your patient. What are his favorite foods or favorite kinds of foods? Then experiment, experiment, experiment. And remember spices! Used lightly, they can change the taste of things and usually for the better.

Twenty-five years ago, the only cookbooks were from Betty Crocker and Better Homes and Gardens. There were no cookbooks written for the patient with diabetes, heart disease, high blood pressure, cancer, ulcers or any other life threatening disease that I ever found. Today, there are many cookbooks and a lot of them are for specific problems. The American Heart Association and The American Diabetes Association put out some excellent cookbooks. Other sources are product suppliers who provide cookbooks with diabetic exchanges using their products. Other cookbooks and magazines will sometimes give diabetics or heart patients an alternative with the recipe. And remember scratch cooking is the best. There are no hidden ingredients when you cook that way.

Check with your local bookstore in the cookbook section. Most offer a good selection of low or fat free, low or salt free, and low or sugar free cookbooks. Try the recipes that more closely correspond to something the patient likes and will eat. Buy products your patient will eat. Now they even make a fat free and sugar free ice cream. Take time to look around and be aware of what is offered. As medicine has made more advances in knowledge about various diseases, the companies that supply foodstuffs have kept that knowledge in mind and now offer a lot of prepared items for the special patient. Just be sure to read the ingredients and know what's in it. If you don't know what an ingredient is or the amount that can be used, call your local hospital and speak to the dietician or nutritionist. They will know or they will find out and they are glad to help.

Mark the recipes they like now and try variations to help them keep liking the food. Their tastes will change. A person who doesn't like soup now may find a few years down the line that soup is all they want to eat or at least a mainstay of their diet. The disease will affect their taste buds. Something they don't like today might be enjoyable in a month or two. Certain medications affect the taste buds and the stomach, and some will give a certain metallic or bad taste to everything. In these instances, you will be better off to offer a variety until something can be eaten without too many problems. That's better than making the buffet line circuit.

Keeping track of things that affect taste will help if and when the medication is discontinued and/or resumed at a later date. It may sound like a lot of hassle, but it's cheaper than throwing food away, or letting the patient not eat at all.

For yourself, as a time saver, try cooking double amounts and freeze them for the days you are sitting in some clinic or doctor's office, returning home too late and too tired to cook.

For about twelve years before we moved to El Paso, we belonged to an HMO, provided by Jerry's place of employment. When we started with the HMO, it seemed better because they were trying to take care of things with medication. And they weren't putting Jerry in the hospital all the time. That made him happy. We thought it was better care; that they were "catching things in time." When we arrived in El Paso, we discovered that he was eligible for Veteran's Administration care because he was blind. Within three months of leaving the HMO, he had two strokes.

When we moved, Jerry was taking forty-eight pills a day. There were seventeen different kinds of pills. The doctors at the HMO were masking the symptoms with the medication. If we hadn't moved when we did, he would have died very shortly. Thank God, I had him for another seven years.

We later learned that the HMO doctors were given certain amount of money for patient hospitalizations. What they did NOT use by the end of the year, they got to divide among themselves. They had an excellent way of keeping the patients towing the line also. If you did anything outside the HMO, you had to pay for it. So much for second medical opinions. If you do ask for a second opinion and get it through the HMO, they just send you to another one of the HMO doctors.

A good thing to do is keep a journal of what medications the patient takes, including strength and amount, what it was for, any reactions, and did it work. Any time they have to go to the Emergency Room, you will have to provide a list of current medications. Keep it up to date and keep it with you. I kept Jerry's either in my purse or in the car. Doctors always want to know what they're taking, especially if the patient is seeing more than one doctor.

Another thing to remember is that most diabetics eat a lot of fruit. Fresh fruit is included in the diabetic exchange and it's good for them. They are usually only allowed so much so you may wind up eating what they can't. Some fruits have very small seeds included. Just a note of interest about seeds, all seeds have a minute amount of cyanide poisoning in them. This, in the seed, is the result of Adam's sin and Satan's work. Don't worry about eating the seeds, though. You could swallow bushels of plain seeds each and every day and it would do you no harm. Just think of all the seeds birds eat.

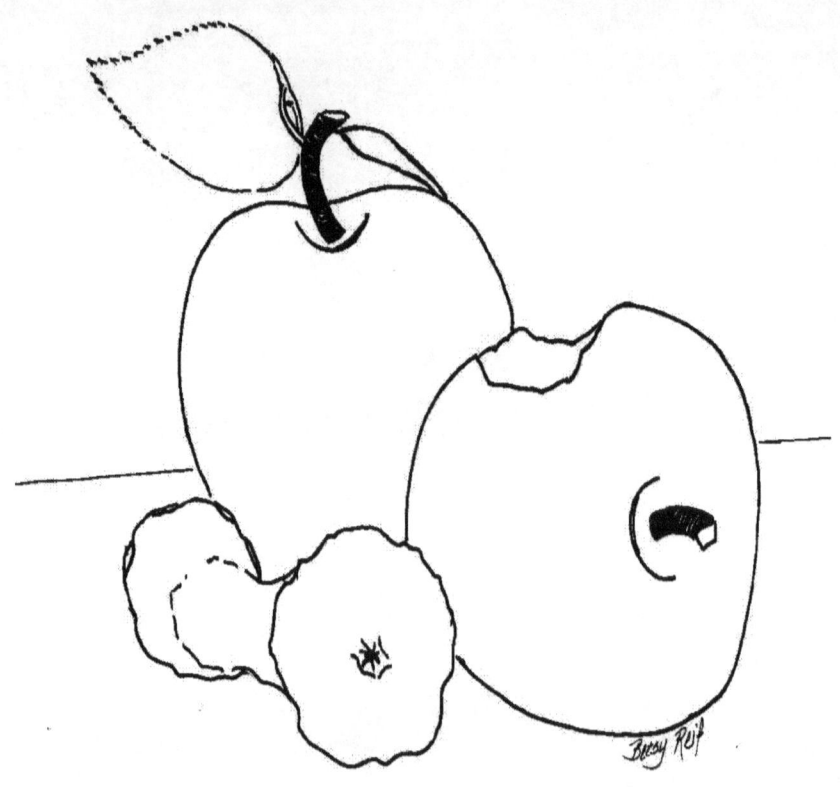

Chapter Four

What Apple? Oops!

A joke from Jerry is always a good way to start.

> On which side of the church should the parents of the
> bride and groom be seated? On opposite sides and as
> far apart as possible. A church is no place to start
> anything.

O f course, as Christians, we know that a church is the best possible place to start things. Many people do not start their marriages in church, but if you don't have Jesus as head of your household, your marriage can very easily fail. There is something about the knowledge of knowing and believing that sometime, in the future, you will have to answer to Jesus for everything you do, especially in your marriage. We may not answer to our spouses, but remember that Jesus sees much farther than spouses. He sees into the heart.

Two examples of wives, from the Bible, to examine in this chapter are Sapphira and Abigail. In Acts 5:1-10 the story of Sapphira and her husband, Ananias, is told. They sold their property and kept back a part of the price, bringing only part of it to lay at the apostle's feet after pledging to give the total amount. Peter knew that they had lied and both of them died because they had lied to the Holy Ghost. They came separately, Ananias first and then Sapphira. But the Bible says she was privy to it. When she came in, Peter asked her why they had agreed together to tempt the Spirit of God and then she died. You cannot lie to God and don't lie to your spouse either, because you can be sure that your lie will find you out.

The second wife we will discuss is Abigail. Her story is told in I Sam. 25:1-42. Now Abigail was a good woman who did the right thing. Her husband, Nabal, was evil and churlish. But because Abigail did the right thing IN SPITE of her husband, she ended up married to King David. Her first husband died when he heard she had done the right thing after he had refused.

Now Nabal was of the house of Caleb, who, with Joshua, had brought back Moses a good report of the Promised Land. But the Bible says Nabal was a man of Belial. He came of good family and surely he must have received good teaching. But he chose to ignore it and made the wrong choice in dealing with David. This shows that you cannot depend on your family, parent, spouse, children, or anyone other than yourself and Jesus, to get you into heaven.

The Bible tells the story of Cornelius, the centurion, in Acts 10, whose whole household was saved. There are many stories of whole households being saved. But even after being saved you make your choice. Sometimes people make the wrong choices as did Nabal. You have to live with those choices, or not live, as happened to Nabal.

Both women knew the right thing to do. But only one did the right thing, and of the four people involved, she was the only one who lived and how she must have lived- married to David, one of the world's wealthiest kings.

How does this fit into care giving? The same way it fits into life. Always try to do the right thing, knowing that God knows the truth and sees into the heart, and right OR wrong there are always consequences- good or bad but still consequences.

The story of Adam and Eve from Genesis, the first three chapters, is excellent for studying the man-woman relationship. Adam was created first, from dust of the ground, and given charge over everything in the Garden of Eden. Eve was created second from Adam's rib. I used to tease my husband saying that men were created from dirt and that's what a lot of them still were. Not my husband, certainly. But of course, women were created from flesh. Somehow, I could never get him to believe that women were better than men.

But God didn't make Eve from a bone from Adam's head that she should be OVER him, nor from a bone from Adam's foot that she should be UNDER him. God made Eve from a rib, one of the softer bones because she was to be softer, a rib from over his heart because Adam was to always keep her close to his heart with love.

Eve was beguiled by the serpent and she listened to it. The serpent said that God had lied to them about eating the fruit of the tree, and that by doing so they would become like God. They would not die. Now, part of Adam's job was to keep the garden and he should have taught her the truth. I can imagine Adam saying, "Don't you touch that tree!" along with "Don't you eat the fruit of that tree." Because that's what she told Satan, "We are not to eat of the tree or touch the tree." (This shows how important it is to KNOW the word of God.) Adam was with her and he saw that she touched the tree and nothing happened. Then she ate a bite of the fruit and nothing happened. So he started to doubt the word of God and ate with her. Ancient Jewish rabbis teach that Adam saw her eat, knew that she was going to die, ate the fruit because he loved her so much that he wanted to die with her. He didn't want to be alone in that garden again.

I have always wondered what would have happened if Adam had not eaten the fruit. Would he have lost another rib for another wife? Would the fact that they were one flesh have been able to save her if he had refused to eat the fruit? Because the word says that it was only AFTER Adam had eaten that their eyes were opened and they saw their nakedness. Adam had watched Eve eat and nothing happened to her so he thought it was safe.

When God came to the garden, they hid. When they finally did come out and admitted to God what happened, Adam said he ate because of the woman. That God had given to Adam. So Adam blamed it on Eve and, ultimately, on God. A friend of mine says men have been blaming everything on women ever since. When God

36

asked Eve why she had eaten, she said the serpent beguiled her. She chose to believe the serpent rather than God. Adam doubted God because he saw that Eve ate and was still alive. You also must remember that death entered the world as a consequence of their sin. I don't believe that they had SEEN anything die before but Adam was supposed to be intelligent and should have known what death was. It was after this that God killed animals to cover Adam and Eve with animal skins. That was the first death in the Garden of Eden.

When God gave the Book of Genesis to Moses, He did not give Adam's reason for doing as Eve did. Perhaps God did not want any of us to agree with Adam.

Also, God wanted people to obey Him because they loved Him, not because they were afraid of Him and what He could do.

One of Jerry's stories to end this section.

A slave was always walking around muttering, "That darn old Adam. It's all Adam's fault. Darn Adam!" One day, his owner heard him and asked why everything was Adam's fault.

The slave answered, "Because he got us kicked out of the Garden of Eden and now we all have to work all day, every day. It's all that darned old Adam's fault.

The slave owner thought about it a couple of days and finally called the slave to him and gave him a closed wooden box that was decorated and very pretty.

"Zeke, I want you to guard this box. I don't want you to look inside, but all you have to do is guard that box."

So Zeke sat around every day, drinking iced tea with his feet up on the porch railing. People waited on him, bringing him meals and tea.

After a couple months, He got to wondering what was in the box that was so important that all he had to do was guard it. He couldn't stand it. Finally, he opened the box and all that was inside was folded piece of paper. He opened it and read what his master had written, "Zeke, I knew you couldn't do it. You are no better than Adam. Now, get back to work!"

None of us could have lived in Eden and left that tree alone. Remember Christmas-time and the lengths some people will go to find out what they are getting as their Christmas presents? Could anyone like that have stayed away from that tree? Sooner or later that fruit was going to be eaten.

We are, first of all, curious and, secondly, rebellious. Every mother knows that. The first word a baby says is "Mama", and the second is usually "Dada". And quite often the third is "No!" If it's not third, then surely it will be in the first five or six words spoken by baby.

I have wondered about the time when the Lord created Adam-dust and dirt being formed into man. Did the Lord look down at His own hands and see the nail prints there? He was the Lamb slain from the foundations of the world. (Rev. 13:8) You and I would have looked at that pile of dirt and wondered if it was worth it. But the Lord did not. This was our loving God that wrote in His word:

> For God so loved the world, that he gave his only begotten Son, that whoever believeth in him should not perish, but have everlasting life.
> For God sent not his Son into the world to condemn the world, but that the world through him might be saved. (Jn. 3:16-17)

To me these two verses should always be given together. For verse seventeen is just as important to me as verse sixteen.

Adam and Eve are the first couple in the world. Love is from God. He designed it, made it and sex. There are many ways to show love and one is to treat your spouse as the most important person in your life after Jesus.

My last job in Milwaukee was coming to an end in November. I had given my notice and the girls all decided to have a going away party. And they were adamant that I had to bring Jerry. They said they just had to meet him. They wanted to meet a PRINCE. Then the story came out.

That spring we had celebrated our twenty-second wedding anniversary. The girl next to me asked, "How can you pick the right guy? How do you know that this one person will stay with you for twenty-two years? There's so much divorce and stuff. How can you know?"

I told her, "Hon, after you have kissed a bunch of frogs, you recognize the prince right away."

She laughed and left and came with the rest of the crew. I had to repeat what I had said. But then I had to finish it. "Now, when you decide that some guy is a frog, be nice. You have to be nice to the frogs because he knows your family and friends. He is going to be somebody else's prince. And it might be your sister, your best friend, or someone you know and want to stay friends with. So be nice to the frogs. Just remember there's a prince waiting for you. Don't settle for a frog when you can have a prince. Then when you get that prince don't ever treat him like a frog. Treat him like a prince and he will always be your prince." On top of that he will always treat you like a queen and your home will be his castle. I found a birthday card for Jerry once that had a castle with a knight on the front and inside a lady wearing a medieval cone hat. Outside it said Happy Birthday to the King of the castle and inside it read from the lady who cleans the moat and feeds the alligators.

Jesus is number one, your spouse is number two, you are number three, your children are number four, your home is five, and way down on the list are jobs, ministries, extended families and further down than that are just friends, bosses, co-workers, etc.

The only one that should be more important to you than your prince should be Jesus, the King of kings!

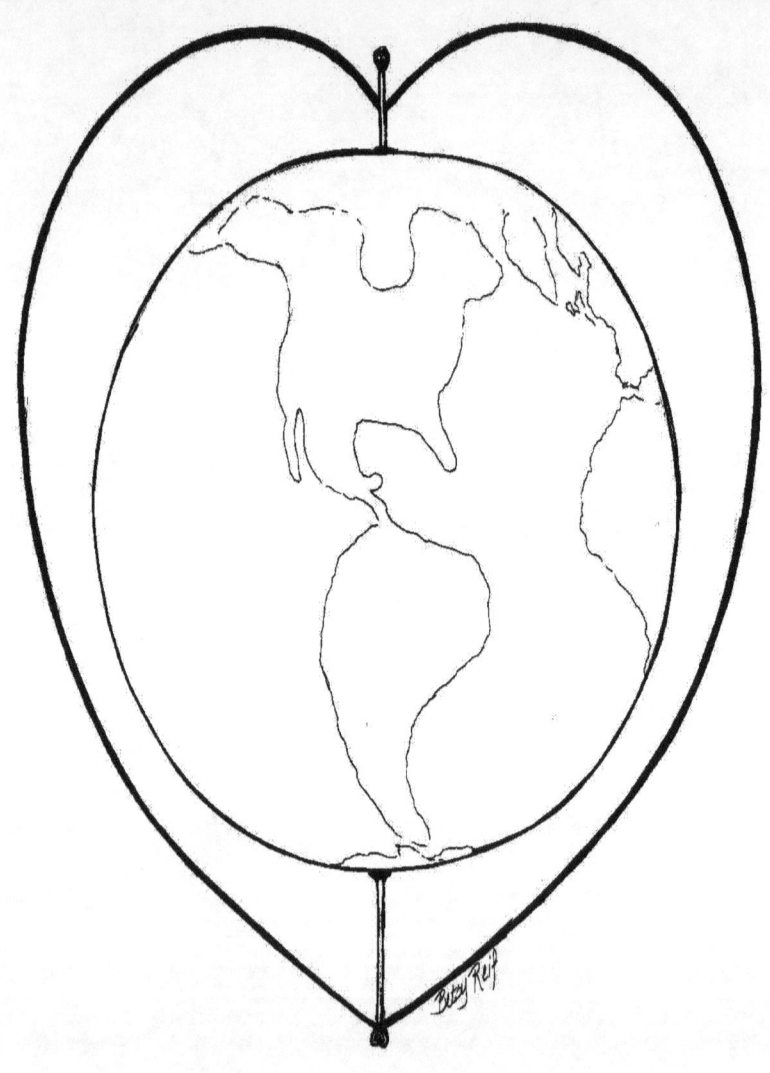

Chapter Five

Love Makes Our World Go 'Round

Love suffers long and is kind; love does not envy; does not behave rudely, does not seek its own, is not provoked, thinks no evil; does not rejoice in iniquity, but rejoices in the truth; bears all things, believes all things, hopes all things, endures all things. (I Cor. 4-7, Nkj)

Jerry and I were happy together. Of course, like everyone else, we had our moments of non-bliss. But like they say, "love conquers all" and we did love each other. And, if you have love, you can survive everything else. The above scripture reference is a description of perfect love. But we muddle along trying our best to achieve it, and when we fail, we must remember that this is a description of perfect love of which only God is capable.

Different diseases have different effects on the body. One of the effects of diabetes is another disease known as neuropathy.

Neuropathy is a disease that affects the nervous system, causing numbness, tingling, or sharp stabbing-type pains in the extremities. One of the extremities of a man's body is his penis. Neuropathy sometimes prevents an erection. This impotence can cause havoc with marital love life. Jerry had this problem, also. Some doctors recommended different implants, and there are several types, including everything from rigid to inflatable implants. There is also medication that can be quite effective but be sure to check on the side effects.

Jerry's solution was not a viable one. He kept saying I should divorce him and go find somebody new who was totally healthy. I told him that was like trading one used car for another. You know what's wrong with the one you have and you don't know the problems you might have with a different one. I had been married before and I knew what might happen.

We discussed everything and all the alternatives with his doctor. He was already sick with an incurable disease and this decision was not one that could be lightly made. It would mean taking chances with something that could cause chronic bladder or urinary tract infections. I was just thirty-five and this was a condition that was going to affect the both of us. I had to make a decision for myself as to whether or not I would be able to live this way for the rest of my married life. It was frightening for both of us.

Then my Christianity began to kick in. After all, I had married him for better or worse. So worse was what came up, but only in one area. His health. After all, it can happen to anybody. There were no promises made. I seemed to remember an old song somewhere, "I never promised you a rose garden." That's true. He had never promised me a rose garden, the moon or any other of these kinds of things. He did promise to love me and take the best care of me of which he was capable. And we did love each other. That was always there. The Bible, in I Cor. 7:5, discusses husbands and wives who withhold themselves from each other by choice and with the consent of the spouse. We did not have the choice but we did consent and chose to stay together.

When the kids were old enough and left home, people would say things like, "Now the honeymoon begins", etc, but I knew and accepted that he could not. I always had to remember that it was not his choice, and that he was not doing this on purpose, but that diabetes caused it and the problem was not my husband's will or fault but fault of diabetes.

Jerry had several healings through the years. He had been golfing in the autumn and, while standing under an old oak tree, an acorn hit him on the top of his head right in the center of his bald spot. (Yes, my handsome husband had a bald spot. You know God only made so many perfect, beautiful heads. The rest He had to cover with hair.) We believed that the point from the bottom of the acorn broke off under the skin. Jerry always said a squirrel threw the acorn at him. He called it being "beaned" by a squirrel. It shouldn't have had that much power just falling. The spot soon grew (not the acorn) into the knot about the size of an acorn. One of our friends called it his knowledge bump because now he was supposed to be smarter than to stand under an oak tree, especially when the squirrels are playing baseball. He had the bump for many years. Then one week, several people prayed for his healing for diabetes, from the top of his head to the tips of his toes. Then a very dear friend of mine, Evie, noticed the bump was gone. Sure enough, he had received a healing. Not the one we were looking for but a healing to bolster our faith.

Jerry started to have problems with his feet. He started to walk sort of flat-footed and looked like an elderly old man getting slower and slower. He had dropped his golfing league so I knew it was very bad. He wouldn't golf even with me unless he took a golf cart. He wouldn't run anymore and had lost the spring to his step.

Our church had a satellite dish, and T. L. Osborn was having a four-day, evangelical healing crusade in Dallas, Texas, at the Word of Faith Church by satellite. On the third day, Jerry started to act a little funny in the service. I worried because, whereas I had read about such healings, neither of us had seen anything like it. It just was not done in our Catholic and Lutheran backgrounds. After the service was over, he wouldn't talk to me but went straight to the back of the church to talk to our assistant pastor. I went to the church bookstore and was crying behind some stacks. A friend of Jerry's asked what was the problem and all that I could think was that Jerry absolutely did not believe or understand what he had seen. So Frank offered to go down and see what was the problem. A few minutes later, Frank returned, a look of amazement on his face. "Maureen," he started, "I'm not sure what all is going on, but Jerry said he's healed!" Sure enough, his legs and feet were healed, instantaneously and completely. He was walking normally.

On the way home, he had to test everything out. I drove past a strip mall and he said, "Pull over." I did. He got out and walked the length of the strip mall. And back. I drove a little further to an on-ramp and he said, "Stop!" I did. He got out and said, "Just follow me! I think I can run!" And he did. All the way down the on-ramp. A squad car pulled up about fifty feet behind me and just stayed there. I know it did look strange, a man running down an on-ramp at midnight with a woman right behind him in a car. I hadn't seen Jerry run for years. He looked like he could have played softball, again. After Jerry got in the car, the squad car still followed us for several miles before turning back. I've always wondered what that officer thought.

Jerry started to feel good enough to try to play golf again. We played a nine-hole course on the shore of Lake Michigan. We always rode a cart and our friends would always take turns with me driving so I could do some walking, also. Jerry didn't walk because he just couldn't see that well anymore. He did well in golf because we would always point him in the right direction, make sure his stance was good and he would make his swing. One of us would always walk ahead and stand behind the flag so he could see us move to it. He couldn't see the skinny flagpoles, otherwise. It always helped him for us to drive the cart straight toward the flag, as we would approach his ball. His legs would get tired so we always tried to make it so he never had to walk very far. He never walked flat-footed and gingerly again and that particular problem with Jerry's feet and legs never came back just as God promises:

> What do ye imagine against the Lord? He will make
> an utter end; affliction shall not rise up the second
> time. (Nahum 1:9)

Jerry started to have different problems with his feet. Diabetic ulcers would appear, first as dark bruises way under the skin. Then they would work their way to the surface as an ulcer- a big open sore. Some were very painful and some he never felt because of neuropathy. But he kept working. He did not receive an instantaneous healing from the Lord for the ulcers. We found a doctor who was finally able to heal them. But it was God who steered us to the right doctor.

We saw one doctor who wanted to cut off his foot between ankle and knee. Jerry refused and God led us to another doctor who used a healing cast on his foot. It healed the diabetic ulcer that was slightly larger than a half-dollar on his heel. I watched that doctor debride the heel ulcer to within $1/1000^{th}$ of an inch to the heel bone. The whiteness of the bone was right there. The doctor said the bone was only covered by a thin membrane. It took six months but it healed.

Jerry also started to suffer from debilitating migraine headaches at this time. They would hurt so badly he would cry. He had some tiny white pills that he had to let melt under his tongue. They were to open the artery in the back of his head. The headaches came about once a month in the beginning. At the end, they would happen several times a day. I felt so sorry for him but didn't know what else to do, but give him his medication and pray.

One Sunday morning, he got a migraine on the way to church. I gave him the pill and said we could go home so he could lie down if he wished. He said no, he wasn't going to let headaches start running his life. So we went to church. Now it was our pastor's way to always pray for the sick at the end of the service. But that morning he stopped right after the praise and worship music. He said that he had a word from the Lord that someone was suffering from a severe headache- possibly a migraine- and that God wanted to heal them and they should just raise their arms. He walked down the aisle toward us. I told Jerry, "Put up your arm!" Because of the pain, he couldn't hear me, so I grabbed his arm and put it up in the air. Pastor Wayne nodded and laid his hand on Jerry and Jerry was instantaneously and completely healed of migraine headaches from then on. Oh, he had regular headaches sometimes, but he never had another migraine. Praise God! Remember the Nahum 1:9 promise.

The thing that other people attest to was his undefeatable sense of humor. No matter how bad things got and some were pretty bad as the diabetes started to rampage, he always had a joke to tell. One of his home health nurses told him that she would tell her other patients about him; how many things were wrong with him and that he always had a joke for her. Somehow, it always helped those around Jerry who didn't know what to say to him.

A little over a year before he passed away, he had a heart attack. I took him to the ER. They wanted to know if they should resuscitate him. I said, "OF course. He was very alive and alert when I brought him in here. Of course you resuscitate him." At two o'clock in the morning they called me. He had had another heart attack and they were going to put him on a ventilator. He was on it for eight days. They keep him drugged unconscious while he was on a ventilator to keep him from pulling it out. But I knew he would recover and get well. Every time he became conscious, he would tell the nurses a joke. One day when I arrived, there were several nurses lined up to ask me what the punch line was because he passed out before he could finish his joke.

The joke always showed them that he didn't want or need their pity or sympathy. He would show them that he was still able to laugh and enjoy life. He would be at ease. He was still the ultimate host caring for those around him. He was running the good race.

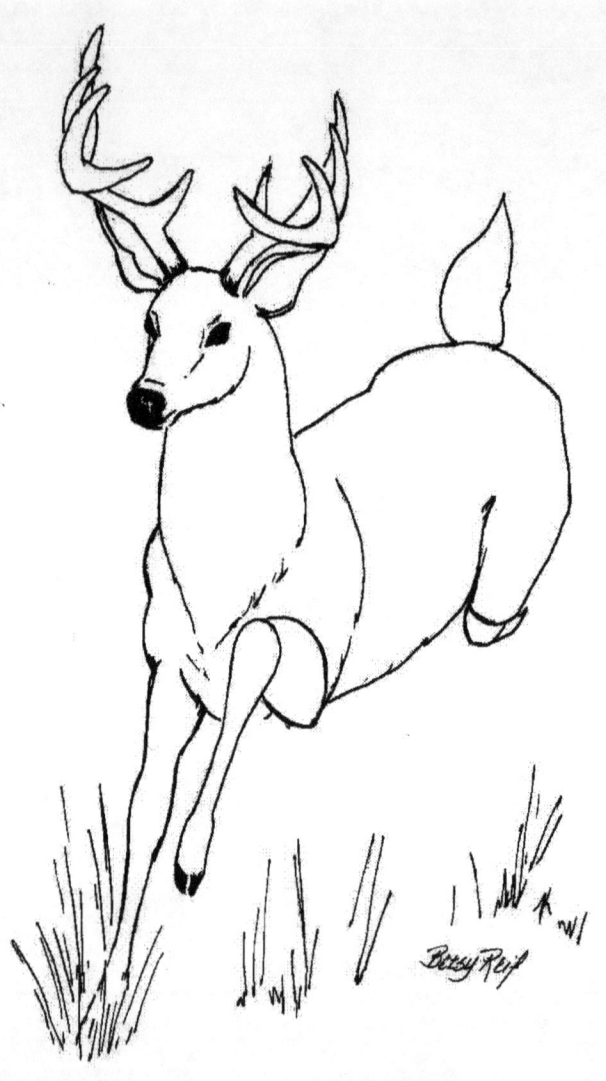

Chapter Six

He Runs Like A Deer

Jerry's joke that fits here:

A city man, driving on the freeway, was passed by a rooster. He wondered how fast the chicken was going so he speeded up and so did the rooster. Again and again until he was going ninety miles per hour and the rooster suddenly took an off-ramp. The man followed and lost sight of the rooster when he turned into a farmyard.

"Did a rooster just come in here?" he asked the farmer.

"Yep," the farmer nodded.

"How can he run so fast?" the man asked.

"Well," said the farmer. "Me and Ma and the boy, we all like dark meat when we eat our fried chicken. So, we experimented until we bred a three-legged chicken so we could all eat dark meat."

"Why, that's wonderful!" said the city man. "How does it taste?"

"We don't know," replied the farmer. "We haven't been able to catch him."

I did finally catch Jerry at the end of the on-ramp but he was never chicken about anything. I think the most important lesson we learned at this time in our lives was the advantage of always getting a second opinion from another doctor. Many people say that they don't like to talk to people who want to discuss their illnesses. BUT because Jerry and I talked to others who had diabetes we were able to change doctors and try other methods. Because of this and the grace of God, we were able to keep Jerry's feet from being amputated for eighteen years.

I believe that with his type of personality and all the things that he enjoyed doing, because he was such an active person, if he had had an amputation, he would have lost his will to live. His survival instincts were very strong, as was his will to live and his spirit of independence.

There are many healing verses in the Bible. I don't know why God did not heal my husband of diabetes. Jerry had received many prayers for healing. Many people, ministries, and Bible study groups around the United States prayed many times for him. In Daniel chapter ten, Daniel was told by the angel that his prayer had been heard the instant that he prayed, but the Archangel Gabriel, bringing the answer to that prayer, had been in battle for three weeks with evil spirits and had to have help from the Archangel Michael. And Daniel was a prophet!

We know that our prayers for his healing were heard and answered the instant we prayed. But there are many evil spirits out there who are very strong and always attack and work against the believers in any way they can. I know there was no problem on God's end. The problem was on this end. Jesus draws the dividing line between the enemies in the Bible very clearly:

> "The thief cometh not but for to steal, and to kill, and to destroy: I am come that they might have life, and that they might have it more abundantly." (John 10:10)

Have you had anything stolen from you? Health? Family? Faith? Anything? Something killed? A relationship? Family member? Love? Something else? How about destroyed? Reputation? Finances? Job? Joy? The thief comes in many ways. He kills. He is a murderer. He lies. He is a liar. He destroys. He is a destroyer. That sounds like an enemy. John 10:10 tells us the thief works against Jesus.

John 10:1 says that he who enters not by the door into sheepfold, but climbs up some OTHER way, the same is a thief and a murderer. Mark 4:15 gives an example of the work of the thief when he steals the word that has been sown into our hearts. And he doesn't stop with just stealing the word of God. He steals anything he can.

We often wonder why do we always feel like we are under attack. The reason is simple. It is because we are. Don't ever be jealous of what the worldly people around you have by thinking that God doesn't take things away from them. That is absolutely correct. God DOESN'T take things away. Satan does. He is the thief. And he doesn't have to attack HIS friends. He only attacks the friends of God. So, if you are under attack, you must be on the right side. Now, just pray up your hedge so strong that when the enemy looks at it, he just says, "There is NO way I can get through it, around it, over it, or under it. I give up."

James 1:17 says that every good gift and every perfect gift is from above and cometh down from the Father of lights. If God gives us good and perfect gifts then how do we loose them? The book of Job tells us how we loose things. Satan tells God in Job 1:9-11 that Job fears God for nothing. That God has established a hedge all around Job and around his house and around all that Job has on every side. In verse 12 God gives Satan power over all that Job has. God allows Job to be tested by allowing Satan through the hedge of protection that God established around Job, his household, and all of Job's possessions. After that, Job starts kicking holes in his hedge by not challenging but listening to his friends instead of God.

This hedge of protection is also discussed in Is. 5:5, Eze. 13:5; 22:30, Ho. 2:6, etc., along with standing in the gap for someone else through prayer. Now we can knock down our own hedge or put a hole in it, and allow the devil to penetrate through our hedge of protection if we have no one standing in the gap. This hedge is very important and the gaps in it are very dangerous. I live in El Paso, Texas, and almost all of the backyards are fenced with rock walls. I know what a hole or gap in that wall can do. We are to prayerfully stand in the gap for those we love and pray for their hedge of protection and our own hedge. As family members, we pray for our loved ones just as all believers pray for their families.

Jerry and I started to notice something while I was attending Bible school. At times, both he and I would see, peripherally, something in the dark shadows that moved swiftly and looked like giant bugs. At first, he would have me chasing around moving furniture and everything else to find these big bugs. (My brave husband was terrified of spiders. I was the official spider slayer in our house.) I could never find them. Then I started to see this phenomenon, also.

I read a book by Dr. Lester Sumrall, discussing evil spirits and how they attack. I began to watch more carefully. I discovered that within a day or two of seeing these things, one of us, usually Jerry, would come down with something such as a cold, fever, flu, etc. Or something would happen such as a close call with danger of some sort. So whenever we saw a giant bug shadow, we would start to pray for protection, casting out and binding up the enemy. It worked. Many times we would find out later what the attack was about but sometimes we did not. We just recognized that God was helping us by letting us see into the spirit realm. Then we would know when we were going to be under attack and that it was time for some heavy duty, all purpose praying.

Then he answered me and spake unto me saying, This is the word of the Lord unto Zerubbabel, saying, Not by might, nor by power, but by my spirit, saith the Lord of hosts.

Who art thou, O great mountain? Before Zerubbabel thou shalt become a plain: and he shall bring forth the headstone thereof with shoutings, crying Grace, grace unto it. (Zech. 4:6-7

Here the Scripture says that the mountain shall become a plain and also mentions a headstone, which signifies the death and end of this mountain.

The apostles were having a problem casting out a demon. They asked Jesus why they could not cast the demon out.

And Jesus said unto them, Because of your unbelief: for verily I say unto you, If ye have faith as a grain of mustard seed, ye shall say unto this mountain, Remove hence to yonder place, and it shall be removed; and nothing shall be impossible unto you.

Howbeit this kind goeth not out but by prayer and fasting. (Mt. 17:20-21)

Jesus answered and said unto them, Verily I say unto you, If ye have faith, and doubt not, ye shall not only do this which is done to the fig tree, but also if ye shall

say unto this mountain, Be thou removed, and be thou
cast into the sea; it shall be done.

And all things, whatsoever ye ask in prayer, believing,
ye shall receive. (Mt. 21:21-22)

Jesus says the same thing in Mark, Chapter eleven. Here we are shown three ways the mountain will be defeated. First, it shall be made into a plain. In other words, flattened. If you're flattened, you have lost the fight. Second, the mountain shall be removed to a "yonder place". That is far, far, away. Thirdly, the mountain shall be cast into the sea. All three methods are very effective for the removal of mountains.

I did a lot of fasting and said thousands of prayers for healing for my husband, but doctors told me that he was doing very well for having adult onset diabetes, having had no amputations and having kept some sight in his right eye for more than twenty-five years.

Sometimes I would lay hands on Jerry or anoint him with oil and we would pray. We saw a few healings- pains, headaches, cramps, and small things. And sometimes he would pull away and say, "Stop. Enough now." And I would have to stop.

In all honesty, at those times, I would think of a double minded man. This also became apparent after he received eligibility for Social Security for Disability and we moved to El Paso and away from his old job. He asked me once what would I do if he WAS healed and his Social Security stopped because he would no longer be disabled. I told him we didn't have to worry because very, very few doctors (none of his) believed in miraculous healing or would admit that they had been wrong (setting themselves up for a lawsuit because of a missed diagnosis) and Social Security wouldn't know what to do about it because of the separation of church and state that they adhere to so ardently.

5. If any of you are deficient in wisdom, let him ask of the giving God [Who gives] to every one liberally and ungrudgingly, without reproaching or faultfinding, it will be given him.

6. Only it must be in faith that he asks, with no wavering- no hesitating, no doubting. For the one who wavers (hesitates, doubts) is like the billowing surge out to sea, that is blown hither and thither and tossed by wind.

7. For truly, let not such a person imagine that he will receive anything (he asks for) from the Lord,

8. [For being as he is] a man of two minds- hesitating, dubious, irresolute- [he is] unstable and unreliable and uncertain about everything (he thinks, feels, decides). (Jam. 1:5-8, Amp.)

This can be one reason a person does not receive a healing. Another reason (not necessarily for healing) but why prayers are not answered is discussed later in the book of James:

Ye ask, and receive not, because ye ask amiss, that ye
may consume it upon your lusts. (Jam. 4:2)

Remember David and Bathsheba? If a man sees a beautiful
woman (or a woman sees a handsome man) and asks God to give
them that person for a mate, and that person is already married, God
will not answer that prayer because that person has prayed amiss. So
that prayer will not be answered. And if you intervene personally you
are setting yourself up for a lot of trouble. If you are ever asked to
pray in agreement with someone for something special and they won't
tell you what it is, don't pray with them.

I have been asked to pray in agreement with people for this
purpose. I have had to refuse. I had one lady who said she just
wanted her boyfriend back long enough to apologize to him. He had
completely disappeared. I stressed I would not pray that he would
stay. I would pray just so that she could apologize to him. Three
weeks later when God answered the prayer and the man came back to
her just long enough for her to apologize, she was angry at me
because he wouldn't stay. In the meantime the man had married. I
reminded her of what I HAD said and how and what we prayed,
THEN she said yes, but that God knew she wanted him back to stay.
God does not read minds. The devil CANNOT and God WILL NOT,
because God is a gentleman. So all you prayer warriors out there be
careful what you are standing in agreement with and ALWAYS heed
a check in your spirit. Be wise! Be smart! Be careful! And for your
sake, be good!

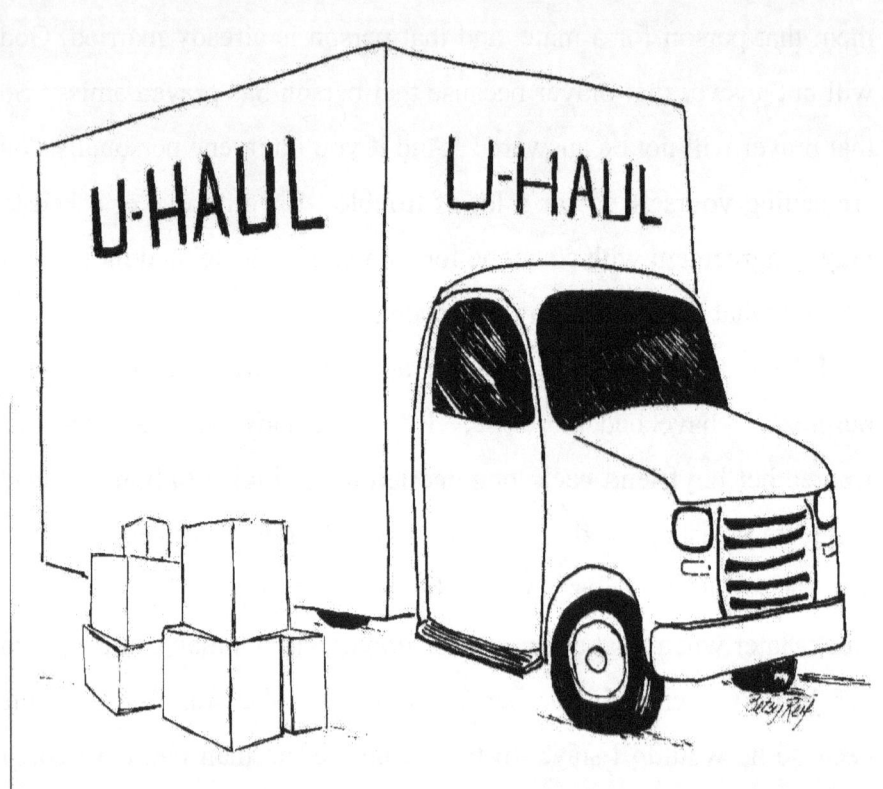

Chapter Seven

Head 'Em Up And Move 'Em Out

A joke from Jerry is in order.

A foursome of golfers were playing behind a very slow foursome. After nine holes, they decided to quit. As they approached the clubhouse, they decided to complain to the golf pro.

He apologized and said that he should have warned them that they were behind four blind golfers and that the play could be slow.

One golfer said, "Gee, I feel bad. Let's buy their round of golf." Another said, "Or let's buy their dinner." The third said, "Yeah, I REALLY feel bad. Let's do both." The fourth golfer said, "Buy them nothing. Why didn't they play last night?"

Jerry's eyesight was failing. We still played golf but only with some very dear friends who would help him in many ways. They helped keep track of his ball because he could not. We would make sure he had a good direction before swinging the club at the ball. Then Ralph would go up to the pin because Jerry could not see the flag stick on his approach shots or long putts, but could see a person standing behind the flag. To show exactly where the cup was, someone in our group would always stand with their feet around the cup. This helped to show Jerry where the hole was. As soon as he made his putt, they would step away. His game was actually improved because he was not tempted to lift his head in order to watch the ball. He could finally keep his head down on his tee shots. But best of all, he was spending time outside, which he enjoyed, playing golf with friends that he loved.

We also went to neighborhood baseball games and all the church games. I usually gave a running commentary on the game because he couldn't follow the ball. We would take munchies and go. One time we even ordered pizza for our supper and had it delivered to the ballpark.

Jerry was declared legally blind and applied for Social Security Disabled Benefits. He got them and less than a year later, in February, he completely lost the sight in his left eye. He just woke up one morning and could see nothing but blackness. This was a very scary time. He was very despondent and I worried about his mental health. There were so many things he couldn't do anymore. He had to give up woodworking, painting, golfing, and yard work. About the only thing he had left were his jokes. I tried to keep my eyes closed for a very short period so I could experience what he was experiencing and I couldn't do it. I couldn't truly imagine how things were for him. Sometimes he would be angry and say something like, "I wish you had this and then you would know what it's like." Then immediately he would realize what he had said and say, "I'm sorry. I don't mean that." I would tell him he had better pray I stayed healthy because who could we get to take care of BOTH of us.

We had friends from church that would come and stay with him or take him for coffee or lunch. Our church family was wonderful. But he always worried that they would get tired of doing it and then I would have no breaks from his care. He thought we should move to Texas where it was warm in the winter and he had family who could help with his care. They even said they would be willing to help.

Jerry could still see moving shadows with the right eye. A few months before that, he had been adamant about being able to drive. He had a midweek doctor's appointment and I had a class. He was so sure he could do it that I gave in. It was a beautiful bright sunny day. He made it fine. But God was protecting the both of us. On Saturday afternoon, we went for a drive and I stopped behind a car making a left turn. He demanded, "Why are you stopped in the middle of the street? You're going to get rear-ended!" I looked at him and was astonished that he couldn't see the car ahead of us. He could not see that car until it started to move to complete its left turn. His trip to the doctor was his final time behind the wheel. We both knew he couldn't drive again.

Jerry had several laser treatments in both eyes. It was kind of new but he could have had it sooner. It might have saved more of his sight or at least postponed his blindness.

That fall we decided to move to El Paso, Texas. Jerry had been briefly stationed at Fort Bliss when he was in the army. He had liked the weather- much different from Wisconsin. And besides, he had a brother and sister living there. His sister had recently moved form Wisconsin, also.

But Jerry had never been around his younger brother, who had retired from the army. He said he wanted to finally get to know his younger brother. We talked to all of them by phone. I thought I could hear a reservation in his brother's voice, so I asked if it was all right, as if we must get their permission to move. His brother said he guessed it was, as long as I didn't pound religion in his head. He proudly announced that he was an agnostic, and if he ever did decide to go to church it would be his wife's church. We later found out that his wife would only go to church once a year at Easter and only IF her mother happened to be in town. I couldn't figure out where they would get the idea that I would pound religion in their heads. I didn't do that to anyone. My born again experience was very precious to me. I only shared it with people whom I loved and with whom I wanted to spend eternity.

After Jerry had been healed of the migraines, he had wanted to share the experience with his sister. So we both told her what happened to Jerry but she, very nervously, just laughed. Later, at their retirement/going away party I was told that I could come to the party but I couldn't say anything about 'religion'. I kept my mouth shut and was subjected to some vulgar jokes about certain television evangelists who were in the news at that time. Jerry was disgusted because it was his brother-in-law and nephew telling the jokes. I had my reservations, but kept them to myself. My husband wanted and needed to have a chance to spend time with his family.

Anyway, we moved. My good friend, Evie, a realtor, sold our house for us and our church family helped us to load the U-Haul truck. Jerry had just finished with a laser surgery in his eyes and was not to bend over or lift anything over ten pounds. I asked one lady from the church to take him and pick up our VCR at the repair shop, his shoes, and other odds and ends before we left Wisconsin. She was able to keep him away from the house almost all day.

We experienced several miracles during this time, especially the sale of the house and God's protection and travel mercies while moving the weekend before Thanksgiving. We had believed that God had sold the house for us at the first open house. So when we got the date and time for the papers to be signed for the closing, we went ahead and got ready. We arranged for the truck rental, utility turnoffs, and people to help us load the truck. I had everything packed that I could. The buyer still didn't have his financing but we didn't know that.

We planned to park our loaded truck overnight at the U-Haul lot, stay overnight with Evie and sign papers the next afternoon. Evie and her broker were both born again, spirit filled Christians. So we got together to pray that night. The broker was having a real problem that we had actually moved out our furniture, shut off utilities, closed the house and prepared to leave the state when the buyer didn't have all his financing.

Anyway, we were all sitting around the kitchen table. Laughter started trying to bubble out of my mouth. I couldn't hold it back. I saw the balconies of heaven with all those people watching in amazement and shaking their heads that we had believed the house was sold and we had operated in faith for two and a half months, only to begin doubting the night before the closing. I moved over into Holy Ghost laughter. I couldn't stop long enough to explain what I had seen. It broke up the prayer session and we went to sleep. The buyer's financing came in about two hours late. We went back to the house to pick up Smidgee, our cat, ate supper at a restaurant, put our car on the trailer, and left town in the rain before it turned to sleet. God is NEVER TOO late.

We had put money down on a house here, sight unseen. I knew the floor plan and it was close to Jerry's family. Anything else could be changed.

It took three days to drive the truck to El Paso. We left Milwaukee at 6:30 Friday night ahead of an ice storm and arrived in El Paso at 3:15 Monday afternoon.

After we outran the ice storm, the weather was good. Jerry and the cat slept most of the way. I stayed awake by singing my favorite Christian songs. The truck engine was so loud we couldn't hear the radio.

By the time we got to southern Illinois, I was ready to stop. I looked over at my sleeping husband just in time to see something on fire fall out of the sky and land about two hundred yards away in a farmer's field, setting some dried cornstalks on fire. I woke Jerry up when I yelled. He said we should go tell somebody. I thought it would burn itself out. Besides, I didn't want to go any place where I could have trouble turning that truck around. I didn't know if it was a meteorite or space junk and, if there was more coming, I wanted to be somewhere else. I simply thought it would be more prudent to just get the heck out of there. That's when it really hit me that the ones I loved the most were in that truck and all our possessions were right there with us.

I wore my white straw hat with navy band because I couldn't find a box to pack it in. Across Illinois, Missouri, Arkansas, and Texas, truckers in their big rigs would pass us because the diesel engine in our truck was not that powerful. I think we prayed our way up some of the bigger hills with angels pushing all the way even after I had geared down.

At Love's truck stop, we stopped to fuel up because I couldn't pass up a place with a name like that. The lady at the register said she was glad to see us. She said several truckers had told her about the woman in the white straw hat, driving a big U-Haul pulling a car on a trailer and that she should watch for us. There were all looking out for us and wanted to know where we headed. She was surprised to see my blind husband and the cat. Jerry and I both believed that, on that trip, we were surrounded by lots of angels all the way.

I didn't have any trouble staying awake or alert. I was tired. Moving is exhausting work. So many things had to be done before we left. We had to have all Jerry's doctors' reports in case something happened on the road. We had to have all our prescriptions refilled so we wouldn't be caught without medicine in case we lost it somewhere. We needed an ice filled cooler for Jerry's insulin. Bank accounts closed, address changes made, so many things to do and you're always afraid you're forgetting something important. But God was with us all the way and I praised Him for His protection. It is scary when you move like that, because you have everything you own with you, including your money. We traveled with a certified check from the sale of our house.

It was about 11:00 p.m. and we stopped for fuel in Odessa, Texas. Jerry was hungry, so he went inside with me. Outside, I noticed a car parked in front, two young men in the front seat and two older men in the back seat. While we were getting our snacks, the two young ones tried to buy beer without the proper identification and the cashier refused to sell it, telling them she would loose her job and the business would loose its license. They walked out very angry and yelling. I went to pay and had to cash a hundred dollar traveler's check. One of the older men had come in, had a twenty-four can box of beer and stood right behind me. He saw into my wallet, easily, and heard me ask about a motel. I was very uneasy.

We stayed inside for maybe fifteen minutes, hoping they would leave. They didn't. We walked to the truck and I helped Jerry in and walked around the truck, still hoping they would leave first. They finally drove to the exit and then WAITED until I drove up behind them. Then they went under the over pass and turned left up the on-ramp onto the freeway, going west. As soon as they were out of sight, I turned right and stayed on the frontage road, going east. We went back to the previous underpass, to cross under the freeway. On the way, we saw the same car now coming east and speeding. I didn't get back on the freeway. Then we saw the same car going slower but still on the freeway and now going west. I told Jerry I didn't like the looks of it and we should stop for the night. We saw the same car come back east again down the freeway and then west again.

I had not been paying attention and wound up on the frontage road dead-end. At midnight, Jerry was outside telling me how to turn the wheel so that I could back the trailer and truck and make a U-turn. I had turned the headlights off so Jerry had a chance of seeing without the headlights blinding him totally. He told me how to turn the steering wheel to keep me from dumping the trailer with the car in the ditch. There was a street light there.

I looked at the freeway and there was that car again, going east very slowly on the freeway. I got Jerry in the truck and went back to the motel that I had missed. I went inside to register and was asking about police patrols for the parking lot when the guard came in. He was an off-duty police officer. He showed us where to park out of sight but under light and promised us he would watch very carefully.

Our room had an inside entrance. We took our snacks and Smidgee, our cat, and settled in for the night. In the morning we heard that the officer had called the police department and had a squad check the car. I don't know what happened to them and I don't know why they were doing what they were doing. That incident was the only time I was afraid of people on the whole trip. But, again, God's protection is everlasting. The next day, we drove into El Paso.

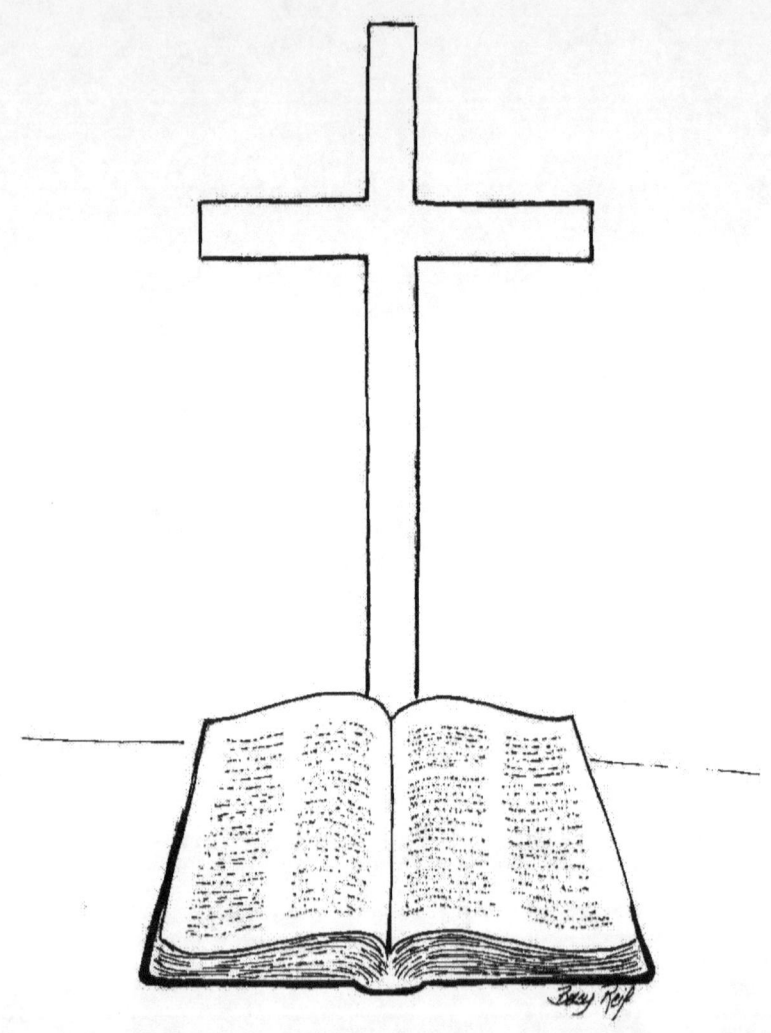

Chapter Eight

Forgive Us As We Forgive Them

We need one of Jerry's jokes to get started.

> A blind man walked into a department store with his Seeing Eye dog, went to the middle of the store and picked up the dog by the tail and started swinging it in a big circle over his head.
>
> The store manager came running up. "Sir, sir! You can't do that with your dog. Can I help you with anything?"
>
> "Oh, no," came the reply. "We are just looking around."

Jerry enjoyed sitting outside in the afternoons or evenings, if it was hot. He was doing some walking with a cane and I'd usually carry a lawn chair in case he got tired and had to sit down. His doctors said to walk and then rest because of his heart bypass surgery. After his heart surgery, he started to have seizures. They are very scary if you haven't seen one before. I was positive he was going to die.

After the first seizure, Jerry's brother came to us and said his wife did not want Jerry to come to their house again. She didn't want her house to have all the paramedics in it if something happened while Jerry was there. Someone told us that perhaps she didn't want to be around a sick person. I had to tell them that that was not the problem. They still came uninvited to our house every night after they finished work and after we had eaten supper to eat our leftovers so they wouldn't have to cook. It also meant that we couldn't do anything after super until after they left.

One day I had made Jerry's favorite supper, baked pork chops with mushrooms and wine sauce gravy. I always doubled the recipe because Jerry liked it and the leftovers. The next day Jerry was expecting pork chops again and was very upset that there weren't any left. That evening, when his brother and wife came again, expecting to eat, Jerry said, "No, we are just on our way out. We are going to a ball game." That was the end of their freeloading.

Jerry enjoyed baseball very much. He liked everything from Little League to the majors. I would hear about people who were handicapped who were not allowed or taken out by their families. I didn't feel that way. I took Jerry to anything and everything he felt he wanted to go to. Hot air balloon races, air shows, the shopping trolley to Juarez, Mexico, out to eat, art exhibits, the zoo, the museum, art galleries, shopping, church, new things to go see like Carlsbad Caverns and White Sands National Park. We went to Montana for my brother's wedding. I tried to keep him on the go as much as he wanted and was able, and to keep him interested in life. I didn't want him to vegetate.

Just remember always to check out the bathroom facilities for wheelchairs if needed. I always took Jerry into the Ladies restroom. He was blind and couldn't see and women are supposed to go inside the little cubicles and shut the door. No one can see them. I thought it was better than for me to take him into the Men's restroom with men using urinals in full sight. We only had a problem one time. A woman came in and saw Jerry while I was inside a cubicle, she went back out saying very loudly, "There's a man in the women's john!" She complained to the woman manager of the restaurant. The manager came in and said that when we came again, we would have to ask for the male busboys to help Jerry in the Men's restroom.

I asked if any busboys were trained on how to help a handicapped person get from the wheelchair onto a toilet and who would be responsible for any injuries. She didn't say anything so I went on and told her that if they should drop him, I would sue and windup owning the place. My first action would be to fire her. She asked us not to come back. We didn't. Some patrons came to us and told us on the way out that we were right and that I should not let it stop me from taking him out to eat.

One time I took Jerry to get his hair cut after he had spend several weeks in the hospital. He always went to the same barbershop. They were good about letting him stay in his wheelchair instead of trying to get into the barber's chair. The barber finished combing his hair and said, "There! He looks good enough to go dancing. You better take him out tonight."

At first I said, "I suppose I had better." Then, like I had thought it over more, I reneged. "No, I better not. I take him out looking out like that and one of those good-looking young chicks will take him away from me." They all cracked up laughing, especially Jerry. Be willing to do anything to keep their spirits up.

The first time the paramedics came, there were people all over. Jerry's brother strolled in and tried to pull me back. I guess he thought I was in the way. He didn't realize that the paramedics wanted information and to see certain things, like his medication and the machine to check his blood sugar. I sort of jerked away from him and got what the firemen wanted.

At the hospital, the doctors came to me and said I had better tell Jerry's brother about diabetes. It seems his brother was telling the doctors that I was doing things to my husband to try to kill him; that I wanted a divorce and that the doctors should look him over real good. This was at an army hospital. This happened twice but I didn't tell Jerry. I didn't want him upset.

The doctors told me that by law they should call the police because a charge by a family member had been made and, then IF Jerry had died at that time, I would have been arrested and put in jail for three days until the police had investigated the charge. I was lucky that Jerry soon regained consciousness and was able to tell the doctors that I had not mistreated or been mistreating him in any way.

His brother said to me that he could find out anything about Jerry's health because he still had friends on the base and at the military hospital. I thought that if he could SEE Jerry's records he could also change them.

I took my concerns to officials at the VA and they told me that if anyone was ever caught letting anybody see official medical records they would not only loose their jobs but be eligible for court martial. No one would risk that.

But I wasn't sure, so the next time he had a seizure, I had the ambulance take him to a civilian hospital. Again, the same thing happened. This time the doctors called the hospital's social worker to talk to Jerry alone. He answered all the questions about his care and how I was treating him. Finally, he asked why they were asking those kinds of questions. The social worker told Jerry what his brother was claiming.

Jerry was furious. I had never seen him so angry. When he found out what the consequences would be for me, he tried to think of all kinds of ways to protect me. Neither of us could imagine anything worse than being put immediately in jail for three days upon the death of a spouse. Some doctors just laughed and told us his family was watching way too much television. We finally went to an attorney and, with his advice, wrote a letter to Jerry's brother. Jerry said he was aware of what his brother was saying and that it was not true, and that if he didn't stop, Jerry would sue.

At that time, we started to be barraged by obscene telephone calls. It was such a problem for us that we were given caller I.D. from the telephone company two weeks before the system was operational. That, and a new unlisted telephone number and some other things the telephone company did, stopped the problem. I suspected it was his brother because during one phone call, I blew a Marine D.I. whistle into the phone as loud as I could. Less than a week later, Jerry's brother had to go to Albuquerque to be fitted for double hearing aids. Somehow his eardrums had burst.

I went to visit a Christian neighbor lady one day. Jerry liked her husband and we were friends, not CLOSE friends, just friends. As soon as I walked into her house, she started right in on me. "Maureen, how can you call yourself a good Christian woman when you are trying to divorce Jerry. To take all the money and just leave him with nothing, how can you do that?" (There wasn't any money.) "That poor man has been through enough. What kind of person are you and how can you call yourself a Christian. Christians don't divorce Christians," and on and on.

I was so astonished that I couldn't even answer her right away. Finally, I got my voice back. "Betty," I said, "Where ever did you get the idea I'm divorcing Jerry? Whoever told you that is wrong. If I had wanted to divorce him I would have done it years ago, not after twenty-three years of marriage." I just sat there. I didn't know what else to do.

Finally, she admitted that Jerry's brother's wife had the idea that I wanted to divorce my husband.

I had enough of the lies and backstabbing. But I didn't know what to tell Betty. After all, she had lived on the same street with

80

them for probably fifteen years. I said that my sister-in-law did NOT like me. "Oh, no," Betty retorted. "She likes you. She says she really likes you and admires you!"

I was so flabbergasted, I didn't know how to respond, but I finally told her, "Betty, if she really liked me, she would not talk about me the way she does." I just sat there for a while.

Betty thought for several minutes without saying anything. I was very uncomfortable and was just about ready to go home when Betty said, "You know, Maureen, you're absolutely right. She wouldn't say the things she says if she really DID like you."

Other things happened that caused a final break in the family relationships for my husband. His sister got involved and sided with his brother. She came to our home and fought with Jerry, saying some very terrible things to him. He blamed his sister for all our problems with his brother and his wife. Jerry said that we had never been around them at all. But that we HAD been around his sister and her husband in Wisconsin.

She pushed her way into our home that day, shoving me backwards out of the way, into the corner of the pool table. I received two herniated disks in my back.

I always believed that she would apologize to Jerry. That is why I never tried to sue her for personal injury. I didn't want a lawsuit between the families to hinder their friendship if she would apologize someday. She never did.

From then on, my back got steadily worse until four years later I could not take care of him at home. Jerry knew it was because of my back injury I had sustained at the hands of his sister. He said he would never forgive her for doing that to me. In the end it affected him, also. He always said he wanted to live at home and die in his own bed. When the officials decided that because of my back injuries I could not take good enough care of him anymore, they decided that he had to go into a nursing home. He hated it. We both hated it.

After Jerry's third stroke, he had problems speaking and eating. His left side was affected with his sense of balance. They were feeding him at the hospital with a tube through his nose. He kept accidentally pulling it out and had his food in his sinuses and I was getting worried. He lost a lot of weight but he refused to eat the hospital food. He didn't like it. It was tough, undercooked, and didn't taste good. Besides, he was being served chicken every day and sometimes twice a day. He said he wanted me to check him over for pinfeathers.

I finally went to the doctor and got his permission to bring food from home for Jerry to eat rather than have him go back on the feeding tube. His relatives started the rumor around the neighborhood that they saw me go out to eat every day but never saw me bring home a carryout for Jerry. Most of the neighbors laughed because they all knew that Jerry was in the hospital (for three months that time) but no one would tell them and the neighbors knew that I was carrying food to him because he refused to eat the hospital food. The relatives tried to get the neighbors to believe that Jerry was inside the house and I was starving him to death but the neighbors knew differently. It took awhile but he made an almost complete recovery from the stroke.

I have told you about families and some of the problems it is possible to run into with them. Not everyone has families like this. Many families will offer to help care for a handicapped family member and will do a super job of it. Some won't.

Some people at a certain moment will offer to help, "Call me," "Just let me know," or "I'll help." But when you ask, they always have an excuse. If you don't want to help someone who has full-time care of a handicapped person, don't offer. Sometime that caregiver will need help and will call. People who have full-time care of a handicapped person need breaks. It is very unhealthy to never get one. Medical people will tell you that that is the primary cause of "Granny Dumping".

Our former church family and friends gave both Jerry and me breaks. When we moved to El Paso, his family had said, "Sure, we can help." But never would.

I contracted the two places in town that were supposed to take handicapped persons for a day, giving the caregiver some free time. One place, run by denominational church, said he was too handicapped to take for a day. Another place, I think it was run by the city, said his Social Security payments were too high. All the time we lived in El Paso, I never got a break from his care except when he was in the hospital or nursing home or that one-day I was in the hospital. In that respect, I regretted moving away from our friends and church family.

Just before Jerry died, I talked to him about forgiving his family. I stressed the Lord's Prayer where it says, "Forgive us our sins as we forgive those who have sinned against us." (Mt. 6:12) At first, he said no, he didn't want to have to fight with them. He was too tired. I said all he would have to say was, "Father, I forgive them." And he finally did. I knew I had to try to do something about the bitterness in his heart toward them. I told him it didn't mean he had to see them or talk to them. Just that he asked God to help him forgive them so that God could forgive him. He did. We never discussed it again.

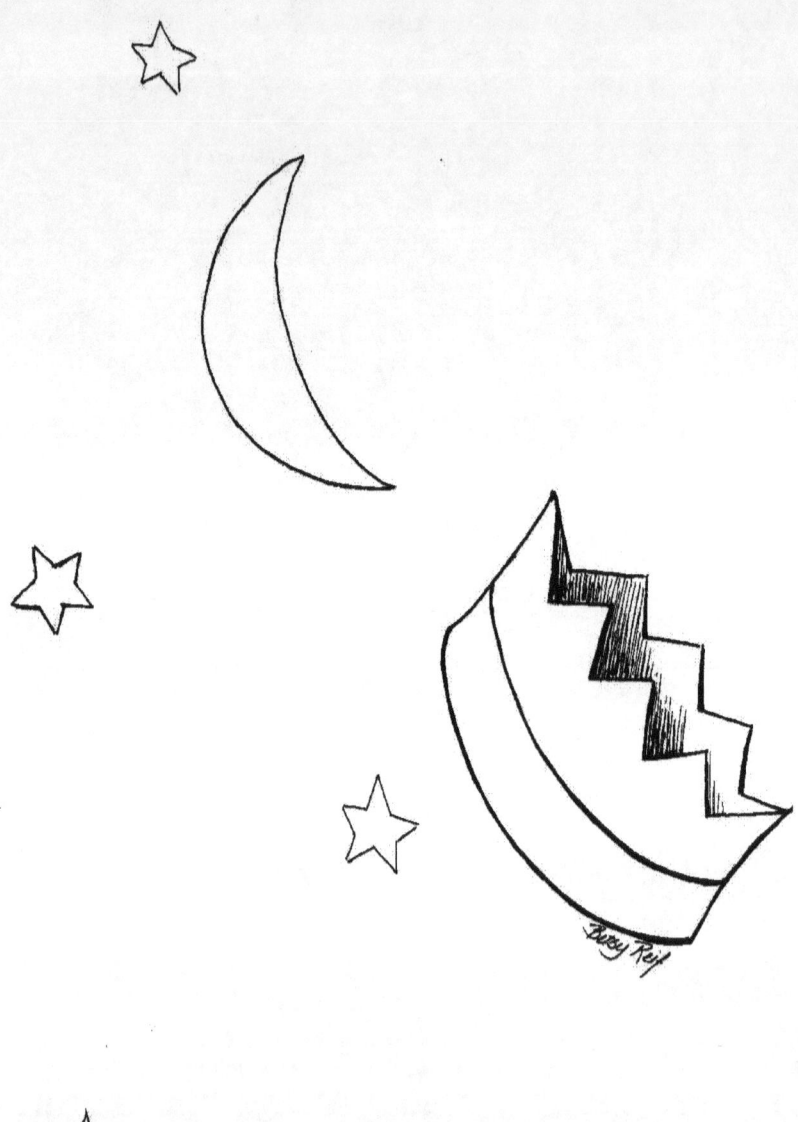

Chapter Nine
Goodnight, Sweet Prince

We must begin with one of Jerry's jokes.

There was an older couple, and one day the man died and went to heaven. About three weeks later, his wife died also and went to heaven where she met her husband. He was showing her around heaven and she couldn't get over how beautiful everything was. The air was so pure it was like breathing perfume. The flowers were glorious and weed free. There was no dust or dirt anywhere. The temperature was warm and comfortable. There was no garbage or trash anywhere. Everything was clean and it was wonderful.

"Everything is just so wonderful and beautiful," she gushed. "Oh, honey, heaven is just perfect!"

"Yes," he answered, "and if you hadn't fed us all that wheat germ and granola bars, we would have been up here ten years ago!"

In July, the doctors told Jerry that he must have his foot amputated. At first, he refused and they said there was no hurry; he could take a week or two to think about it. They sent him to a nursing home. We spent everyday together. I would come and push his wheelchair outside.

During the last five years, his neuropathy had gotten worse. He was incontinent and had started with an external catheter and for the last three years had lived with an indwelling catheter. He also lost bowel control at times. He would say, "Honey you should divorce me and find somebody who is healthy."

"Oh, no." I'd tell him. "I know what I got now and I don't know what I would get. I'll keep what I got, thank you."

He would cry and say, "But you shouldn't have to do all this. Diapers and catheters and everything. It's like taking care of a baby again."

"Yep," I'd tell him. "This one weighs more and can tell me where he hurts or what's wrong, that's all."

The attendants in the nursing home would not clean him up and if I made a stink about it, they would give me the clean stuff and tell me that if I wanted it done, do it myself. So I did.

The attendants in this nursing home stole food from his tray or said he could not have it because he was a diabetic (never mind that a dietician had ordered it for him). He was constantly hungry. Again I was taking food to him. I would read the menus and couldn't understand why he would be so hungry.

So I went one day just to watch. I saw attendants tell patients, "You've had enough," and remove the tray. Or if a patient complained that they didn't like one item on the tray, they would say, "Well, you must not be hungry," and they would remove the whole tray. Jerry was blind and they all knew it. I also saw them slip containers of food into their pockets. This nursing home was investigated by the state of Texas after one of their patients starved to death and the doctor turned them in. The man in the other bed in Jerry's room was never fed food all the time that Jerry was in that nursing home. When I mentioned it I was told that the man's Medicare had run out and he and his family had decided to withhold his food because there wasn't enough money to pay for him to stay there. He and his family wanted him to die.

I was ready to sign Jerry out and take him home when he said he was ready to have his surgery.

I was scared and didn't want him to have it but they said he had dry gangrene and a very good chance of getting regular gangrene. After that, I also wanted him to have the surgery. Gangrene of any kind is scary. I knew the surgery was a must.

He went into the hospital and, in September, they removed his left foot. He was in the same room for several days with a man who had pneumonia. From there, he went into a rehabilitation hospital. He had a fever and they thought it was an infection. He came home

Christmas Eve. He was trying to eat and to take care of himself whenever he could. January first I took him back to the emergency room. He was not allowed to come home again.

Finally, the injury to my back had become bad enough that I had to give up my cane and walk with a walker. It was hard to get around and extremely hard to take care of Jerry.

He had lost weight. He weighed 180 pounds but was still too heavy for me to lift and he couldn't help enough. The state of Texas said I was no longer able to care for him and they put him in a nursing home. I went to a rehabilitation hospital as an outpatient for treatment and after my treatments I would go see Jerry. I would read to him and play the piano for him. We would listen to music tapes or teaching tapes.

While he had been in the military hospital, they had severely scraped his foot on a metal chart holder that hung on the foot of the bed. The nursing home (another one) couldn't heal it so they sent him to the wound care center. The doctors there admitted him back into the hospital.

Something happened while they were debriding his foot. They never told me what. He was in the cardiac care unit but, when I saw him, he was black and purple from his waist to his upper thighs, all the way around his body. I was sure this was blood. It was too huge to be a bruise. Somehow they had punctured a blood vein or something. Of course, they never admitted anything was wrong. But from that time on, every other day, he had to have a dialysis.

God gave me a vision of Jerry while he was in the hospital. I don't know whether or not I was awake or asleep. I saw Jerry naked with no sores or scars or black and blue marks on his body, standing tall, on TWO feet, laughing and able to see with TWO eyes. He had all his teeth and lots of hair and he was smiling and laughing. He looked so strong and tall, standing there waving his arms and clinched hands over his head in joy. I was so happy. I went and told Jerry what I had seen and that I believed God was showing me that He was going to heal him.

Jerry started to cry. "Maureen, did God REALLY tell you that he was going to heal me?" he asked. I told him to remember that healing is in the Word. We cried together.

Much later several people that I mentioned the vision to told me that they knew then Jerry was going to die and they believed that God was showing me that He was going to heal him- in heaven. How happy and healthy Jerry would be then.

The dialysis was very hard on him. It made him extremely tired. Sometimes he would tell me to just go home; that he wanted to go to sleep.

About this time Jerry started to see someone dressed in white in his room or walking into his room with me. He would ask me who was there with me or who was standing on the other side of his bed or somewhere else in his room. This happened several times at the hospital and a lot at nursing home.

I saw his father who had been dead for seventeen years go into the intensive care unit when they chased me out into the hall. I also saw a woman sitting on the corner of his bed. When I described her to Jerry he identified her has his mother. I didn't tell him I saw her next to him but I made out like I had seen her in a picture at some time or other which I had not.

Finally the hospital said he was well enough to go to a nursing home that had a critical care unit. It was supposed to be a step down from the hospital. They moved him on a Tuesday. Monday he had had dialysis. They never gave him dialysis again. I was told that that the reason the hospital sent him to that nursing home unit was because they had their own dialysis machine. Unfortunately, they had no one on staff who could run it and had to hire someone to come in especially to run it. They didn't always have the funds to do that. But I never discovered this until much later.

At first, they had him way down the hall. He couldn't use a bell and they couldn't hear him. They kept the door closed because they said he had lobar pneumonia. The pneumonia didn't surprise me too much. While he was in the military hospital, just before Christmas, the other bed patient had pneumonia. After New Years, when he went into the nursing home, the other bed patient went to the hospital TWICE with pneumonia. Most of the staff wore gowns, masks, and gloves when in his room.

I would come and find that he hadn't eaten; no one wanted to feed him. He needed help with trays because of the blindness and the neuropathy. He couldn't open containers, remove plastic wrap, cut up his own food, open sugar or salt packets, or even hold his silverware to feed himself.

He now weighed 160 pounds. I came one day and found food all over his bed. They just left him with the tray and, when he tried to feed himself, he upset it. Another time, when I asked him why his food was all over his bed, he said they pushed so much food in his mouth so fast that he couldn't breathe. He had to spit it out so he could get a breath and the attendant said, "If that's what you're going to do, you don't get anymore." I know several days he had nothing at all to eat. I knew how sick he was because he didn't asked me to bring anything from home and when I offered he just said no, he didn't want anything.

They didn't want to change his bed if he messed it or do anything much for him. They kept him tied in bed, both hands and his foot. When I would come I'd complain about it. They said he kept pulling out his feeding tube. "With his foot?" I'd yell. I always let him loose and as soon as I left they would tie him up again. He hated lying on his back and he was forced to by being tied.

There was a nurse stationed outside his room but the door was kept closed. Monday afternoon I got to his room and heard him groaning and moaning in pain. The nurse just looked at me and said he had been doing it all day. I started to open the door and she looked in and grabbed the door and shut it in my face.

"We have to get him cleaned up." And she went in and started calling on the intercom. People started hurrying in but they wouldn't let me in. Finally, I just walked in. Jerry had fallen out of the bed with his arm caught in the bedrail. Yes, the bedrails were all up and somehow he had fallen out between the bedrails and the entire weight of his body was suspended on that one arm, putting pressure on the shoulder joint. They took X-rays to check for damage. I always thought that he had tried to walk.

That day, they decided to move him to a room closer to the nurses' station. It was about eight thirty that night when I left. I didn't get to kiss him goodbye because he was surrounded by staff. It was the only time I didn't kiss him goodbye. Going down the hall I started to cry. For the first time ever, I told God, "If You are going to take him, take him quickly and don't let him suffer anymore." On the way home, I came over the crest of the hill and I saw a rainbow so close that the end of it was just a few blocks way. I would drive through it.

At a quarter after ten the next morning, they called and said they were taking him to the hospital. I asked if I should hurry or if I had time to shower and change clothes. The nurse said to take my time; there was no hurry. As she hung up, I heard her say, "Geez, I hate making these calls. You never know how to answer them." She was disgusted.

I got there at eleven a.m. and asked the emergency room nurse which cubicle Jerry was in. The hospital chaplain came up behind me. "I'm so sorry, Mrs. Schulz."

I took one look at him and started to scream and cry, "NO, NO, NO!" They got me out of the waiting room. I asked to be taken to him. He had tubes in his nose and in his mouth and was so cold. I wondered how long he had been dead. The chaplain asked if there was anyone he could call for me. I told him I had a list in the car and

94

someone got it. He made all the calls for me, collect so I didn't have to find money for them. I had already made arrangements with everyone to call them periodically, collect, so that Jerry could talk to them from the nursing home.

At one point, the staff all left me alone with Jerry. I thought to myself, "I don't accept this. I went to Bible School and I had learned how to bind up the enemy and cast him out." I started praying and just as I was starting to bind up and cast out the spirit of death, I heard a still, small voice inside me say, "Look at his body. He doesn't WANT to go back." I stopped and started crying all over again.

Remember when I talked about Noah and where was God? Inside the ark. This voice said, "He doesn't want to GO back," not "He doesn't want to COME back." The voice was where Jerry was, not where I was. We both believed in healing and raising the dead because we had both seen it. We had seen healings of both the deaf and blind. One man we knew was supposed to go to the dentist. He was terrified but after much prayer, he went. The dentist asked who had filled the man's teeth. The dentist said he hadn't seen work like that. The man's teeth had not been filled with dental cement, they had been filled with silver. A parishioner died of a heart attack during Sunday morning service. Some nurses and paramedics in the congregation took him out into the hall to lay him flat and do CPR because he wasn't breathing and his heart had stopped. The pastor laid hands on him, anointing him with healing oil. An usher called the ambulance and everyone in church prayed for him. After about twenty minutes, the ambulance came. But the patient was already breathing and trying to talk and sit up. Both Jerry and I had seen too much not to believe.

After I had been sitting there with Jerry's body for about an hour they said I must call a funeral parlor; that they had to get him out of the hospital. The chaplain even made the arrangements for that and the cremation, everything. The man was wonderful. I later wrote to the hospital and told them how much he had done to help me and how much I appreciated it.

They didn't want me to drive home alone. I had no friends or relatives that I could call on. I finally asked him to call a neighbor. She picked me up and took me home. Shortly after I got in the house, the nursing home called and asked if I could get Jerry's things. Later, after the neighbor's husband got home from work, we went back to the hospital, he drove my car home and she and I went to the nursing home to pick up his belongings.

That was the end of the most horrible day of my life. My sweet prince was gone.

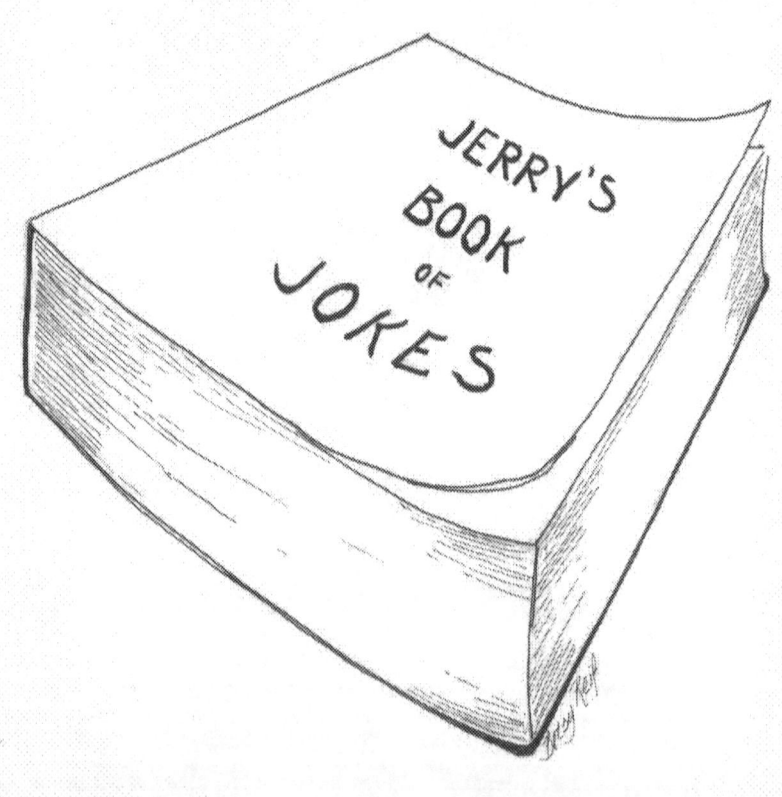

Chapter Ten

Return To God

THE PROMISE

by Maureen Schulz

I can not hold you anymore

Because you are gone.

The voice that soothed and comforted me

I cannot hear.

The face I love, the smile that touched my heart

The beautiful eyes, so blue so clear

The arms that cannot hold me

Hands that will not touch me again

Have gone away from me.

I am so alone and cold.

The love I have for you remains;

We shared so much,

Two lives twined together into one.

I am empty now, ripped apart.

I curse you, Grave,

And I will hate you, Death forever!

I am left alone with this promise.

I love you, sweetheart,

And we will live together, again,

In heaven.

Heaven seems a long way away when you have lost a loved one. You know in your head that they are now with Jesus in a better place with no pain or sadness. And your heart clings to the fact that their spirit is alive and that someday you will be together, again.

Jerry and I had made a decision years before to be cremated. Neither one of us wanted to make the other have to take care of a grave or go to a gravesite to feel close. While Jerry was in the hospital and nursing home, I had begun searching for a church to attend. We tried to go to church when we first came to El Paso. We went to different churches. Finally, Jerry didn't want to even try to go anymore. People would let their young children come and stand around Jerry and stare at him. They stared at the wheelchair, his tubes, his blind eye, until he felt like he was on exhibit. He'd whisper loudly, "Maureen, get me out of here!" We would go.

I had narrowed the field to only two churches. I contacted one and asked if the pastor would hold a memorial service for Jerry. There would be no casket or graveside service because he was being cremated. The pastor said he would but he did not believe in cremation. He cited Joseph asking that his bones be taken back to his father's land when the Hebrew children left Egypt (Ex. 13:19). It was four hundred years later and his bones should have turned to dust. He had probably been mummified for his bones to last that long.

But my problem with what that pastor said was if it was necessary to carry Joseph's bones back, then why not all the other people that had died during those four hundred years? I believed that it was a personal request that Joseph made of his kinsmen and that's why they did it. It was not a request made by God. In reading and studying the word of God, you always have to carefully discern between what God says and what someone else says. If only people who are buried are allowed to go to heaven then why will the sea give up its dead? (Rev. 20:13) When they say 'ashes to ashes, dust to dust,' ashes are even mentioned first.

So I went to the other church and one of their pastors said they had no problem with cremation and that yes, I could have a memorial service for Jerry in that church without being a church member. I believe that there should be more teaching on this in churches to help people make decisions before it's necessary. They teach us how to live and we believe that the spirit NEVER dies. Why not how to handle the death of a body?

It bothered Jerry that we had not found a church to join after moving to El Paso. He asked me if I would say some words over his body after he had died. I said yes, I would. While he was at the funeral parlor, waiting for the autopsy, I went and asked if I could see him. My cousin and her husband were with me. At first, the funeral director said no, I could not see him so I started to leave. I got as far as the car when I said I could NOT leave. I had to go back and fulfill my promise to Jerry. When the funeral director realized I wasn't going to leave, they finally let me see him in a storeroom.

He was on a gurney but they had removed the tubes from his nose and mouth and had cleaned his face. I read the twenty-third and ninety-first Psalms, Ecclesiastes chapter three, and 2 Corinthians chapter four. It gave me peace to know I had done as he had wanted. Also, it made me feel better to see his body without all the signs of the trauma he had endured when they tried to resuscitate him at the hospital. He looked peaceful.

I made phone calls to tell everyone who should know. I told them that he was in heaven now, with Jesus, and he wasn't suffering anymore. One of Jerry's relatives, a Jehovah Witness, told me, when I said he was with Jesus now, rather loudly that he was not. He was dead. God mercifully did not let me hear any more. She spoke several more minutes. When she stopped I told her that I believed that he WAS with Jesus because that is what MY Bible said and I chose to believe that and said goodbye. After that encounter, I had to spend some BRPT (Bible Reading & Prayer Time). I just opened my Bible to the middle hoping for the Psalms and my eye fell to a verse that God, in his mercy, showed me at that time when I needed it so desperately.

> Then shall the dust return to the Earth as it was: and
> the spirit shall return to God who gave it. (Ecc. 12:7)

My daughter said very coldly, "See, Mom. All that praying you did didn't help, did it?" I never tried to explain to her that we must all die once only, (Heb. 9:27), regardless of what the people who believe in reincarnations believe.

My cousin and her husband had a music ministry at some churches and nursing homes where they live. Jerry had heard them sing and had some favorites. I asked them to sing three of the songs he liked; 'When He Was On the Cross, I Was On His Mind', 'Where the Timbers Cross' and 'Serenaded By Angels'. Then everyone sang, How Great Thou Art.

I went to Wisconsin three weeks later and we had essentially the same service. There were more people who had known Jerry for many years attending the service in Wisconsin. The Pastor's eulogy was different because this pastor had been personally acquainted with Jerry for a number of years. He said he gave Jerry a good report as pastors are required to make a report.

Different ones read poetry or told how Jerry was remembered by them. Many mentioned his sense of humor and good attitude in the face of adversity and ill health.

The man who sang was the son of the couple we had golfed with for years. He was a pastor and singer, but he didn't know the songs. He had twenty-four hours to learn the songs, and God was with him because he did a great job.

I had written a poem for Jerry while he was in the hospital one time and it meant a lot to both of us. I read it at both services.

103

Memories

by Maureen Schulz

Memories, wonderful memories

That I have with you,

I won't be sad, I won't be blue

While I have these memories I share with you.

Memories of what we've done

Lots of good times-we have had fun.

And all the best things we have found

Are in our memories and keep us bound.

Memories are what age is made of.

Good memories feed deep, abiding love.

I hear you snore and I'm not alone.

You're beside me and we are home.

Memories that we have built

Can cover me like a cozy quilt.

Make me feel safe, keep me from harm

And when I'm cold, they make me warm.

"With this ring, I thee wed."

Those were the words that you said.

"Until death we shall not part."

I've hid those words deep in my heart.

The days have gone, the years have passed.
But memories are the things that last.
They can't be stolen, they can't be sold.
Worth more to me than silver and gold.

Whether you're here or gone from home,
With these memories, I am not alone.
So, I'll collect memories and hold them near
And I want you to know that I love you, dear.

After I returned home, I had to start to find a way to survive. I applied for Disabled Widow's Benefits for Social Security. I also applied for a number of jobs. Because I was disabled and walked with a walker no one wanted to give me a job. Some even said, "You're just too handicapped." Or "I don't believe you will be able to get around here without falling. It's too dangerous." (They didn't want me to fall on their premises and then sue.) Only one employer wrote me a letter thanking me for considering them and making an application. Social Security said I could still type. I can- about twenty words per minute, (but with only one finger). I can't sit too long and have to stand up and move around every hour. Now, three years later, I cannot stand.

I found that one of Jerry's insurance companies screwed up. They only had one column to list the beneficiaries in the one column but he wanted me to be his beneficiary if I was alive, and if not, then our three children were to share equally. That's not how the insurance company did it. They made my share equal to the children. I only got a fourth to pay medical bills. I didn't have funds to pay some bills. So I advise EVERYONE to have your insurance company SHOW you how they have listed your beneficiaries. One misunderstanding can hurt the person who has to pay the final bills. Make sure you know the status of every policy, whether lapsed or paid up.

Jerry always told me that his policy through his International Union was for $5,000.00. When I sent in the request for it, and talked to some union members, I was quoted everything from $3,000.00 to $700.00. I did not receive a check for $5,000.00. It was less than $2,000.00. But I didn't have paperwork for it. The union had it.

Each state is different, but for federal records I also advise all caregivers to pay themselves a salary out of the other person's social security check. You will be paying into social security yourself then, and it won't look as if you were unemployed for years on end.

Well, this book started out to be a handbook for caregivers- those people who have full time care for another person, usually a loved one. That was pretty dry reading. And there were many things that I had to explain why I was saying them. Finally, I changed it to just telling our story. If you are smart enough to be a caregiver, you are smart enough to spot the things that gave us problems and how to avoid them. I tried to share Jerry's jokes enough to lighten up what could be some very heavy reading. If it helps anyone, then I am glad. Perhaps Jerry's favorite television shows could do a show about caregivers and help many people out there who are truly the Good Samaritans of today. May God be with you.

God gave us a three-part blessing because God is three persons in one, and because we are created in His image, we are three part beings. The three persons of God are Father, Jesus, and the Holy Spirit. And they do all exist separately and at the same time. Mat. 3:16-17 shows this. Gen. 1:27 says we are created in His image, not a monkey's image. We also have three parts; body, soul, and spirit (I Thes. 5:23). The three-part blessing is Nu. 6:23-27 (NASR).

23. "Speak to Aaron and his sons, saying 'Thus you shall bless the sons of Israel. You shall say to them:

24. The Lord bless you, and keep you. (This is for the body)

25. The Lord make His face shine on you, and be gracious to you; (This is for the soul)

26. The Lord lift up His countenance on you, and give you peace.' (This is for the spirit)

27. "So shall they invoke My name on the sons of Israel, and I then will bless them."

Verse 23 commands the blessing. Verse 24 is for the body of man. It says "bless you" (the body of man). To "keep you" and that means taking care of you as Adam was commanded to "keep or take care of" the Garden of Eden. To "keep" is to feed them and that is

107

possible because of the food of God the Father has put on the earth. Verse 25 is for the soul of man. It says the Lord will make His face to SHINE on you. That's showing His glory. (Moses was not allowed to see the face of God in His glory, only his back parts Ex. 33:18-23. In verse 20 God says, "You cannot see My face, for no man can see me and live.") When our bodies are dead and our spirit is alive and in heaven, then we can see God in His glory. He will make His face to shine upon you. And who can miss the graciousness of the Holy Spirit, the third person of the trinity. Verse 26 is for the spirit of man. It says," may the Lord lift His countenance on you." Countenance is "face" without showing His glory. When God is angry He turns AWAY from people. Psalm 60:1 asks that God turn BACK toward his people again. Jesus says He will give us His peace (Jo. 14:27). We can have peace in our spirits and live in peace if we subject ourselves to do the will of God and follow his commandments. He promises to lift up His countenance on us and not turn away from us.

This is from God the Father who loves His children enough to give them guidelines for living in His blessings. All three parts of man are blessed in the three part blessing that God blesses us with. Some churches use this blessing to end their services. So I ask, may God bless you in this- His own special way.

I guess they wanted to hear brand new jokes from a new joke teller in heaven. Maybe now he will put all his jokes down in a book for all those in heaven to enjoy. Jerry was absolutely sure he was going to heaven when he died. Some people are not sure that they will go to heaven when they die. If you want to be sure you will go to heaven, the following is a short prayer for salvation.

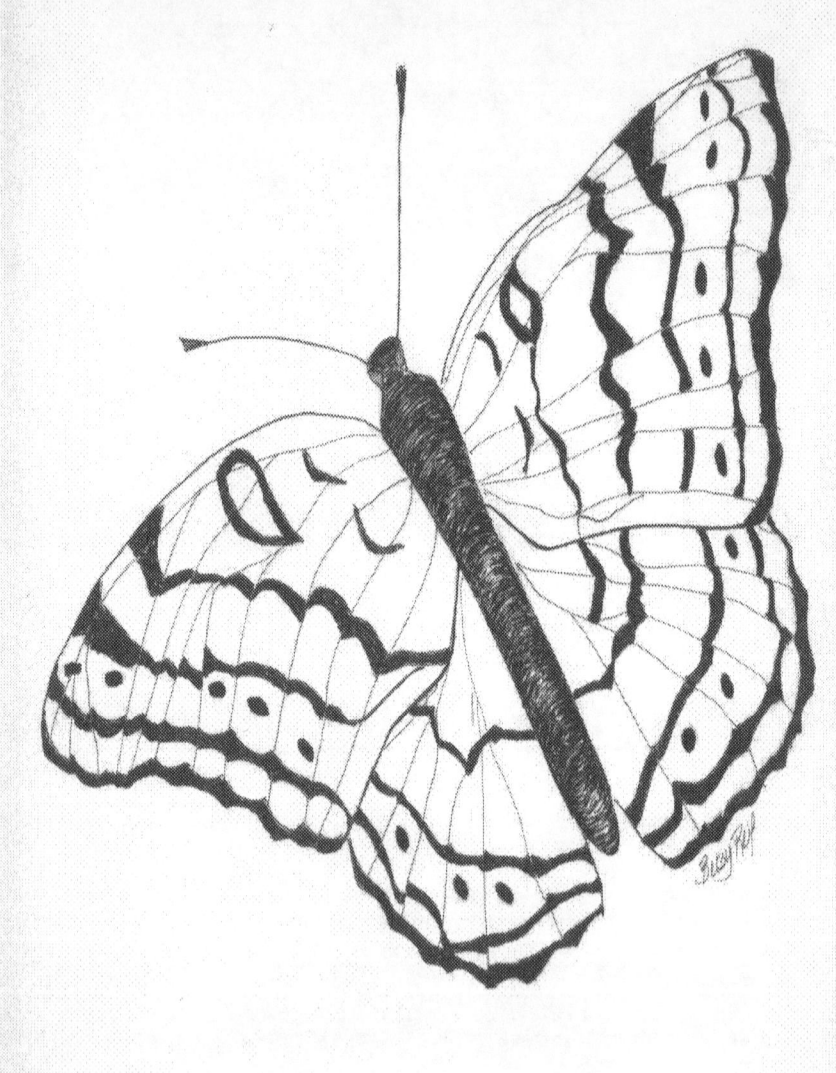

PRAYER FOR SALVATION

Dear heavenly Father, I believe that You created heaven and earth and all things. I believe in Jesus Christ, Your only begotten Son, who was crucified, died for the remission of our sins and was buried, descended into hell, on the third day He arose and ascended into heaven. Lord, I ask You to forgive all my sins, to come into my heart, to cleanse me and be my Lord and Master for ever and ever, Amen.

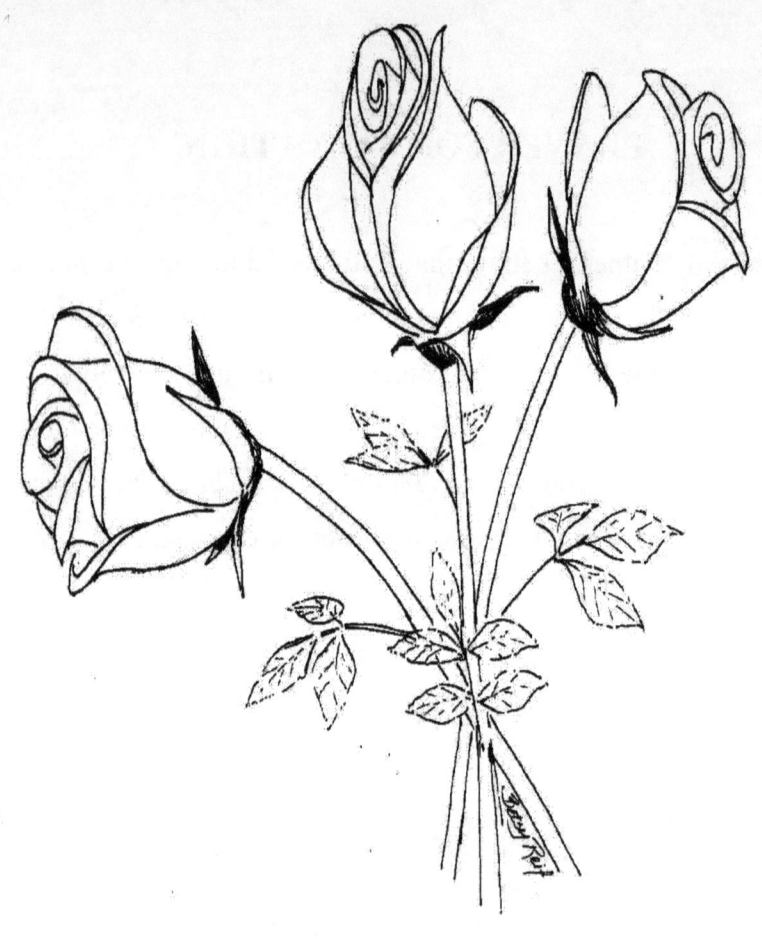

ROSES

by Maureen Schulz

The rose petals are drifting down.
The fall leaves are dying all around.
They're free now blowing along the ground.
The stems no longer hold them bound.

The summer green I thought so dear-
The lovely colors are gone, I fear.
The wind is all that I can hear
For fall is now and winter's near.

The birds have decided not to stay.
The butterflies have flown away.
But they'll be back some warm spring day.
And animal babies will come out to play.

The winter season makes me blue.

My love, I don't know what to do.

My arms ache to hold on to you

But I have nothing to hold on to.

With spring, life comes to a forest glen.

A promise God gives to all men.

My heart will heal with time and then

I'll watch the roses bloom, again.

SUMMARY

The author has written the story of her life with her husband and his battle with diabetes. This book started out to be a handbook for caregivers- those people who have full time care for another person, usually a loved one. That was pretty dry reading. And there were many things that the author had to explain. Finally, she changed it to just telling their story. If you are smart enough to be a caregiver, you are smart enough to spot the things that gave them problems and how to avoid them. She tried to share Jerry's jokes enough to lighten up what could be some very heavy reading. There are many out there who are truly the Good Samaritans of today. May God bless you and be with you always.

ABOUT THE AUTHOR

The author is a retired sixty-one year old widow who keeps herself busy writing, reading, and watching television, especially all the old movies that she never had seen before. She writes poetry and has received several awards.

She lives in El Paso, Texas, with four furry, four-footed feline friends who walk on leashes. J. R., a tomcat, inspects everything and keeps his three sisters in line. Cooney likes to go visiting. Lady Jane is very regal and ladylike and Babycakes spends most of her time sleeping.

She has a stepson in Wyoming, a daughter and a grandson in Connecticut, and a son in Wisconsin. She has traveled a lot in the United States and has many friends.